these are my sisters

these are my sisters

AN "INSANDECTOMY"

by Lara Jefferson

ANCHOR PRESS/DOUBLEDAY
Garden City, New York, 1974

ISBN: 0-385-08442-0
LIBRARY OF CONGRESS CATALOG CARD NUMBER 73–82256
COPYRIGHT 1947 BY VICKERS PRINTING COMPANY, INC.

LIBRARY
University of Texas
At San Antonio

To the "mental surgeon" responsible for my rebirth. During my bloodless "insandectomy" he removed egotism—and left endurance. And to the immortal "Bard of Avon." He replaced inaction with concentration and left—"Shakespearian salvation."

LARA JEFFERSON

INTRODUCTION

MANY YEARS AGO the original manuscript of this book was
written in the violent ward of a state "Mental Hospital."
Whether it came out enclosed in letters or "all of a piece" we
do not know. Penciled on an odd assortment of scrap paper, it
was almost impossible to interpret.

Though it contains many mixed metaphors, split infinitives,
peculiar phrasings and odd similies, we have preserved it in its
original form. We believe it depicts every human emotion in
graphic, meaningful words. Shakespeare himself could do no
more.

Many gripping lessons in psychology and human relations are
set forth, but nowhere is any crusading, any preachments, any
"pointing with pride" or "viewing with alarm" carried on.

Since it was not written for publication, no preface was provided. Because the authoress is unavailable to prepare one, we
must forego any "fiction" and leave it out.

We, the publishers, who could not write a preface or prologue
to it if we tried, submit this book for exactly what it is. We
believe it will be all things to all people. Here, to name a few,
you will find religion, tragedy, pathos, love, truth, jealousy, psychology, sex and insanity.

We could say with Robert Burns:

> O, wad some power the Giftie gie us
> to see oursels as ithers see us.

> It would frae monie a blunder free us
>   an' foolish notions

but we prefer Omar Khayyam when he said:

> The moving finger writes, and having writ
>   moves on: nor all your piety nor wit
> shall lure it back to cancel half a line,
>   nor all your tears wash out a word of it.

We like the dignified simplicity of the radio introduction heard so often a few years ago:

> Ladies and Gentlemen, the President of the United States.

The quiet human dignity of this book warrants the same treatment, so we say:

> Ladies and Gentlemen, These Are My Sisters.

JACK VICKERS,
editor and original publisher of *These Are My Sisters*

these are my sisters

CHAPTER 1

BECAUSE I AM I, an odd piece of Egotism who could not make the riffle of living according to the precepts and standards society demands of itself, I find myself locked up with others of my kind in a "hospital" for the insane. There is nothing wrong with me—except I was born at least two thousand years too late. Ladies of Amazonian proportions and Berserker propensities have passed quite out of vogue and have no place in this too damned civilized world.

Had I been born in the age and time when the world dealt in a straight forward manner with misfits as could not meet the requirements of living, I would not have been much of a problem to my contemporaries. They would have said that I was "Possessed of the Devil" and promptly stoned me to death—or else disposed of me in some other equally effective manner.

But because the poor deluded tax-payers of America insist on the delusion they are civilized, they strain themselves to the breaking point to keep institutions for our care in operation. Then when they break down under the strain of trying to live up to the standards they set for themselves, the officials, whom they have appointed for the office, pronounce them insane—and they are committed to institutions.

I know I cannot think straight—but the conclusions I arrive at are very convincing to me and I still think the whole system is a regular Hades itself. But there is nothing I can do about it—for I have been relieved of the responsibility of trying. It is just another of the vicious cycles that are forever whirling about our destinies. And it is just my hard luck it whirled me into an insane asylum. Here I sit, even though I was one time a so-called intelligent member of society. I doubt that my wisdom had ever great depth or wide scope even though I did make a conscientious effort to live up to the demands of civilization. I must have had a fair share of intelligence, or I could not have conducted myself according to the rules as long as I did. But now I cannot conduct myself as the rules set forth because something has broken loose within me and I am insane—and differ from these others to the extent that I still have sense enough to know it;—which is a mark of spectacular intelligence —so they tell me.

Here I sit—mad as the hatter—with nothing to do but either become madder and madder—or else recover enough of my sanity to be allowed to go back to the life which drove me mad. If that is not a vicious circle, I hope I never encounter one. But today the circle has stopped chasing itself long enough to drop me somewhere along the unmarked line between stark lunacy and harmless eccentricity. The latter is as near to normal as I ever hope to get. I am not relying on my opinion in that matter. The doctor was through just now and flattered the extent of my intelligence and education by discussing me in some long-handled, technical words I suppose were the labels for my phobias.

For all I know of what he said, he might have been swearing at me in Yiddish. But I did get this much out of his very learned discourse—and his face was more serious than it has ever been when he addressed me previously—that unless I learn some new mental habits—and learn them in a hurry one of these days in the not far distant future I am going to find myself over on "Three Building"—and when you land on "Three Building" you have fallen to the very bottom, you are hopelessly and incurably —insane.

Unless I learn to think differently, I shall shortly be incurably insane. There it is before me in words—small, black words, written with one hand and a stub of a pencil—and on my ability to do what he admitted was one of the "impossibles" my fate is hanging.

It is just up to me—the power of the life within me. There is nothing another can do to help me. The job is mine. With all of the study men of his calling have devoted to abnormal people —nothing has been discovered which will enable them to reach into the dim caverns of a crooked brain and make the crooked places straight. They have endless ideas and theories—but when it comes down to actual performance of making an insane person sane—they are helpless. Because I knew something was happening to me that I could not comprehend, or cope with, I came to them for help. In all fairness to them I am certain they have given me the best they had. But madness is like a cancer—it must be treated in time if the patient is to recover. And for me— there is only "Three Building" left. It does not matter.

Life, for anyone, is an individual thing. For one who is insane —it is a naked—and a lonely thing. I learned that in my days of raving. I am aware of it more than ever this morning, as I think of what is before me. Insanity—Nakedness—Loneliness—Hopeless insanity—on "Three Building"—unless I can learn to think differently.

How—how—*how*? In the name of God—How does a person learn to think differently? I am crazy wild this minute—how can

I learn to think straight? Is it after all, of so much importance whether there is one more—or one less—mad woman in the world?—Because I am the woman—and because I have more than my share of egotism—it matters—tremendously—to me. Then there are those who love me of whom I dare not think at all just now. To them—death—that has to do with shrouds and coffins, would be preferable to the chaotic darkness.

But I am morbid—and I caught at this pencil to try to stop my morbid introspection—not to continue it. It was a wild idea—generated in a wilder brain. Nothing can stop my thinking —nor straighten it—and I am headed for the crash—into "Three Building."

Something has happened to me—I do not know what. All that was my former self has crumbled and fallen together and a creature has emerged of whom I know nothing. She is a stranger to me—and has an egotism that makes the egotism that I had look like skimmed milk; and she thinks thoughts that are—heresies. Her name is insanity. She is the daughter of madness—and according to the doctor, they each had their genesis in my own brain. I do not know—and I doubt if the doctors are as sure of what they think they know as they would like others to believe—or would like to believe themselves. I know nothing about such things, at least not in the way their knowledge runs.

They have a list of long Greek and Latin words and when they observe such and such symptoms in one of us, they paste the label for our phobia on us—and that is the end of the matter. I cannot see that they have accomplished so much in merely being able to remember all those long-handled names for our madness. We, who have learned what madness is by going through it,—(and you cannot have closer knowing than that)—are sep-

/14/

arated from all others by a gulf so wide that it cannot be bridged. And there the matter lays—divided, split, and sundered.

Ancient races said madness was "Devil possession"—and dealt with the victim after the manner that suited their time. Their sophisticated descendants, because they live in the present and call themselves "modern," have dispensed with the devil idea—and developed an intricate system of symbols. Words, technical phrases—whose syllables clatter together and make a noise like scientific analysis. They do not have the insight to know that the whole thing is summed up with as much logic in some old voodoo witch doctor's symbol.

But this is getting me nowhere. If I must learn to think differently—there is nothing to do but to go about doing it with what few remaining shreds of intelligence I have. But how—is the question. It is plainly my job for none other can do it. How can I escape the fate stretched before me. The easier way is to let it all slip, and to cease from all caring or trying. But that is not the answer. As long as there is a shred of me left, I dare not do other than try to find some sort of balance between the conflicting forces driving me. It is not a new problem. I have had to contend with it always. It is as old as all of my living—and I still have not solved it. Madness. It has always been waiting before me—behind me—pursuing me.

I was only a child when I first felt its hot breath upon me. In childhood I started down through the years in headlong flight trying to escape that which could not be escaped. And now there is nothing much left of the past but the echoing memory of foot-steps. Foot-steps—fleeing in panic through the years. Foot-steps—whose pattering echo is trampled and deadened beneath

/ 15 /

the earth-shaking tread of the monster—so sure of his prey he could take his own time in the catching.

Those of you who care to, can ridicule the "power of suggestion," you can scoff at the thought of "ideas implanted." I, poor soul can only remember.

I was the child of a woman of forty-six—and a man of seventy. Five children were born to my mother before I arrived. These five and her three previous husbands had died before I was born. All succumbed to some wasting disease, such as meningitis or malaria. The oldest lived fourteen short years. The youngest only a few months.

As my mother went further and further into the menopause, she prayed for a child who would survive. That prayer was answered. Perhaps it shouldn't have been.

Even before conception I was pledged to the service of God. How else than by prayer could a woman of her age and a man of seventy implant these seeds? After my birth my mother's menopause lasted sixteen years, yes,—sixteen years of disturbance —of ill health, of a fanatical fervor that I should be another Mary. That I, the answer, should pay off her debt.

I learned to read, to memorize, to quote from the Bible. My mind was crammed with knowledge no child should be forced to absorb. I was to be an evangelist, to lighten the troubles of the world, I was to lead people unto God.

My mother had, in her younger years, been an attendant at an asylum in a neighboring state. Her suckling children were brought to her at intervals for nursing by a patient who had only to walk across the grounds. Yes, only a few hundred yards across the lawn where even other patients took turns caring for these fatherless children.

As I grew and studied she told me of these days, of the things behind those grey walls. She told me of those poor mortals who had driven themselves insane through sin. Of those who had such a feeling of guilt they could not bear it and sought solace in oblivion.

I, too, was sinful, I was worldly. I could not grasp the feeling that the salvation of the world hinged on me. I wanted to be a girl, not a saint. And mother again told me of those whose thoughts were not saintly—and of their fate.

When she found I would never be a mesmeric speaker, never a direct messenger of the Lord, she decided I should do the next best thing. I should become an evangelistic musician. Through the stirring tones of music the "message" would be conveyed. Three years later she found me tone deaf.

I had debased her before God, I had failed in "My Destiny."

Contempt crept upon her. Downward—ever downward I slid on the scales of her regard.

Finding myself taking refuge in deliberate forgetfulness, in fanciful dreams, in delusions which included no music, no "leading the world into light"—life became easier,—until she sent me to a convent. This place was not unpleasant, but I left it as soon as I could, and went back into the maw of contempt and unkind condescension, back into a whirlpool of misguided mentality, (which could only be exceeded by pulling the plug out of the Pacific). I shouldn't have gone back. Never should I have returned to her repetition of: "The fear of the Lord is the beginning of wisdom; and to depart from Evil is understanding!" I had neither the fear nor the wisdom—only what she thought was the evil. Now I am paying for it.

Whether I had more insight than others, or whether it is a fact that the thing feared by us is the thing which befalls us, I do not know. However it got here, the fact is glaringly present that it did overtake me in the twenty-ninth year of my living. It caught me and swept me—where, I do not know. All the way through hell—and very far into heaven. Now it has whirled and left a stranger unknown to me. Sitting here in my body, I am weak, sick, and vomit much, and stagger so I can hardly walk. At the least movement, perspiration breaks out all over me—I am a fool—and I know it.

The State has adjudged me insane and I am no longer responsible for anything, so it is stupid and senseless for me to try and salvage anything out of the tangle. But since the tangle is I, I cannot let it lay as it is. Even though that would be better—still, I cannot do it. I still have a life on my hands—even though it must be lived out in an insane asylum. Though I have lost every encounter, I am still not dismissed from the conflict. If all my weapons have failed, I must find some others.

I cannot escape from the Madness by the door I came in, that is certain—nor do I want to. They are dead—past—the struggles of yesterday. Let them lay in the past where they have fallen—forgotten. I cannot go back—I shall have to go onward—even though the path leads to "Three Building"—where the hopeless incurables walk and wail and wait for the death of their bodies.

I cannot escape it—I cannot face it—how can I endure it.

The whole thing is a dream and a nightmare. No doctor ever stood before me and told me that I would shortly be incurably insane unless I learned to think differently. Oh, I am sure it is all just a dream. Presently, I shall wake up and be oh, so relieved—to know that this has all been a dream. Then it will be only funny—and I can recall with humor the odd sensation I had on finding that a crazy woman had moved into my body. A crazy woman who had no sense at all, and who refused to be governed by reason—who acknowledged no law higher than her own whim—and who had no fear of anything. I shall shortly awake and remember how frail my strength felt and how helpless I was in trying to budge her gross and unseemly proportions. Dreams seem quite real as you dream them, but how quickly they pass; when I awake I shall be able to laugh at this nightmare. For that is what this great skinned horse is—somebody's nightmare.

She is not real—she is not I—I never saw her before I dreamed her. I am dreaming her now. If I am not dreaming her—then someone else is. And presently they will wake up and this whole thing will dissolve into the night—where nightmares go on waking. Oh, it is all a dream—a delusion—a nightmare. Nothing is real. Everything is a wild toss of hallucinations of one kind or another about one thing or another. All this other raving and howling going on around me—will not someone come and awaken me—so that I may go free?

If I am to be awakened—I must awaken myself—for no one else can do it. But I do not know how. There is only a shadow remaining of the person I used to be. My whole former life has fallen away so completely it might be an existence lived in the Stone Age—leaving only a few uncertain bones to mark its passing. If the person whom I used to be could not prevent the birth of the person I have become, there is not much chance that the latter more powerful creature will be controlled by the ghost of the person whom she succeeded. I attended the death of the first, and superintended her burial. Her casket was a straitjacket and she was buried in a cell in an insane asylum. To others, I was only a maniac—howling—but who, by some odd quirk of nature had the canny Scotch foresight to ask for a strait-jacket before Madness claimed me.

Perhaps a relentless Recording Angel knew what was happening and was able to write it—but I did not understand it. The struggle that followed was waged above—or below—my conscious knowledge. All I could do was to feel—startlingly—nakedly—starkly—things no words can describe.

I was locked away in a cell—stark madness my only companion. The heavy brass lock confining me was nothing more than a symbol. Had I been the sole inhabitant of the most distant star, I could not have been more alone. No—it was not a brass lock which taught me what the nakedness and loneliness of living means. For I have kept a lone death watch with Madness —when Reason was dying.

As Madness attended the death of the first—he also ushered in the birth of the second. Though the nurses released the same body they tied down—the creature who moves about in it is not the same person. Let those who think they have an explanation of such things, explain it. I do not understand it. The whole thing is a dream—an illusion—a tricky arrangement—as slyly drawn lines can confuse the eye when a seemingly straight forward pattern will shift from one thing to another, and the first outline be lost in the second, even as the eye watches.

If it is an illusion—it is none the less real—and if this latter person whom I have become was concealed all the time in the self-same outline as the other—I would rather go through death, than the wild chaos of shifting back to the other. Let the first one lie dead—along with all the other things of the past. I would not call her back if I could. None can write her obituary better than I—for she was I. A pitiful creature who could not cope with life as she found it—nor could she escape it—nor adjust herself to it. So she became mad, and died in anguish—of frustration and raving.

The worst that could be truthfully said of her is that she was a fool and a coward. The best:—that she did have the foresight to see Madness coming, and make grim preparations. She took only herself to destruction. And God alone, who knows all about inner emotions, is the only one able to judge whether her end was a defeat—or a triumph.

I have learned through the grim lesson taught by my failure that my previous methods of trying to adjust to the problem of living were not the right ones. If my wrong way of thinking was the net my mind spun to entrap me, then it is certainly logic, that the same sort of spinning cannot release me now that I am entangled. I do not know what is the trouble—only that something is wrong—terribly wrong. And I do not know how to right it.

There is nothing solid to stand on—nothing beneath me but a vast treacherous quagmire of despondency—followed by periods of exultation and ecstasy; and neither condition has any foundation in logic. All my life I have been either in the throes of the one or the other; and I have an empty, sick feeling when I think of the energy wasted in trying to hold my moods down to something like reason. And now—since Reason has slipped—altogether—and I still have not solved the problem—well, there is only "Three Building" left.—Unless—unless—I can do that, which, if it could be done—would be a miracle.

In the brain of this crazy wild woman, who was born while I lay in a jacket, a crazy idea is turning. Because she was born during madness, the idea resembles the monster who sired her, at least, it seems so to me who used to set great store by reason. She suggests very seductively that the best weapon with which to fight fire—is fire. And suggests fighting madness with madness. Perhaps she is not so insane as I think—perhaps she is saner than I was before she came to me. She presents her idea with so much logic she makes me think that instead of losing reason in madness—and finding insanity on the other side—that in reality, I will lose insanity in madness—and find a sound mind on the other side.

Whichever is right I know that I have been all the way through hell—and found the rest of myself somewhere on the other side. But the part of me that madness led into hell—could not endure it. The fierce heat of the journey consumed the stuff she was made of. She melted away to a shadow. This latter creature has thoughts of her own—and will not be controlled by a—shadow.

If the weak, fearing creature that I used to be, had ability to generate, out of her weakness and fright, such a creature as I have become—then the world must have had her all wrong. She was not an imbecile—but a genius; even though the creature that has grown out of her weakness and failure is a—monstrosity. If a colossal egotism is the mark of a maniac—then she is a maniac—and will shortly be on "Three Building," the prospect does not worry her in the least. She has come out of hell, and has both the odor of smoke—and scorched flesh—upon her; so she has the audacity to look at the fate stretched before her—and laugh—as she sees it. She cares nothing at all for the things that her predecessor considered of value. She mocks at the shadow of her former person—and waves a bold flag of defiance. And I still am divided. I cannot truly forsake all the old ideas as long as their memory stays with me. Neither is it at all likely that I can impose them on to the maniac I have become.

Any creature that can be governed by reason is not a maniac. And this latter creature has a method of reasoning that is not based on logic—but is more convincing. She reaches her conclu-

/22/

sions in a streak that is naked and piercing. She does not rely on the slow process of thinking to reach a conclusion—but cuts a broad swath through the "feelings"—like a streak of chained lightning.

I do not know what to do with her—nor how to withstand her nor to educate her and teach her some of the decencies I was taught at one time—and tried to put into practice. Oh, she will land up on "Three Building"—there is no doubt. But she just mocks about it—and tells me that it does not matter at all whether life is lived inside an insane asylum or out of it.

She tells me that I have missed all the main issues of life— and can see nothing clearly. That I have concerned myself with the externals only, and have missed all the meanings of the great inner significance. That there is no such thing as a normal mind —or an abnormal mind; but only minds and more minds. That life is the important thing—not the classification of it. Life. To live it—and not fear it. Let it rip—let it roar—let it be destructive if it must, but live it and do not fear it.

She whispers that I became mad—not because of some inner deformity—but because of too close supervision and trying.— Trying to force the thing I was into an unnatural mold. I do not know. I doubt if she has the right idea—but if all this latter trouble that has befallen me is a result of too much restriction— then I think I see a new place to apply much restriction— then I think I see a new place to apply the abhorrence we feel for the Chinese custom of foot binding.

All this crooked philosophizing is not solving my problem. Let those who think they know the causes that lie back of disintegration set themselves to the task of evolving an effective treatment in freeing the victim. Or if that is not possible—let those wise enough to think to the root of the trouble, be also humanitarian enough to teach those not so gifted—how to cope with the problem. Finding the cause—or fixing the blame—if it ever is done, will come too late to help me. The fact is, I am already here, in an insane asylum—and in the big middle of Madness; headed straight for "Three Building" and hopeless insanity—unless I can accomplish a miracle. I am already entangled—and if I am freed I must do it myself for none other can help me. And I have precious few weapons—and little equipment—unless Mother Wit, out of my very great need can forge me a weapon to meet the necessity.

Because I must face the problem and deal with it somehow—I evolved this paper and pencil idea. I had the pencil in my hand as the Doctor talked to me—and when he had finished and gone out and left me staring at my hands with stupefaction—the idea came to me born of illusion. I heard the noise of the others tied down in their raving—(one of them is dying and does not know that she dies)—and I felt all this tumult of madness—all this stark, lonely living which is worse than death—and the pain, futility and hopelessness of it all—and the endlessness, the eternity—and the sound became mixed in my brain with another meaning. It was beating and sweeping around me—a flood—released from God knows where—and dashing us all to destruction.

I looked at the others—and felt an odd feeling of kinship. I looked at the strait-jackets that held them—(from my own arms the feeling of being tied has not yet departed)—and the thoughts that came to me then—are between my own God and myself—for they were madness. The flood that was swirling about me was sucking me under—and the pencil I had in my hand was a straw to be caught. It was just a straw—but I caught it—and now I have kept my head above water for a while—even

if what I have written does not make sense to anyone—at least
—it has helped me a little. I have been able to find a few inadequate phrases. And anything that can be whittled down to fit
words—is not all madness.

It is only ideas of such colossal proportions that a symbol for
them cannot be created—that are vague and intangible and
brooding, incomprehensible and fearful, that produce madness.

The very fact that a thing—anything—can be fitted into a
meaning built up of words—small, black words, that can be
written with one hand and the stub of a pencil—means that it is
not big enough to be overwhelming. It is the vast, formless,
unknown and unknowable things that we fear. Anything
which can be brought to a common point—a focus within our
understanding—can be dealt with.

I do have a pencil and enough sheets of paper to last for
awhile—and as long as this crazy woman that I have become,
wants to rave—what matter if the sound of her raving falls into
words on the paper—or goes off into air, and mixes with all
the other tumult and uproar that goes on down here. Her thinking is wild—but I have the wilder idea that if I can force her to
keep it hitched to a pencil, and hold it down to the slow rhythm
of writing things out in long hand—the practice might tame
her somewhat. I would rather try to tame a wild bull in a pasture. I know not how to deal with her because she is a maniac.
Because she is I—and because I still have myself on my hands,
even if I am a maniac, I must deal with me somehow.

The nurse just now picked up one of the sheets I have written.
She read it—looked at me oddly—and asked what in the hell
I thought I was doing. And because she expected an answer in
keeping with my strange occupation—I did not have the heart
to disappoint her. So I gave her an answer that fitted. I told her

that I was Shakespeare, the reincarnation of Shakespeare trying to sidestep a strait-jacket. (I'll admit that I feel queer enough to be the reincarnation of something but I doubt if Shakespeare would claim me). But hurray! She came back down the aisle with a whole ream of paper and said to me: "Go to it, Shakespeare."

Verily, verily, Shakespeare, I had no idea you could be called from your quiet English grave with so little effort. In my present predicament, I know of no one who could be quite such a fortunate choice for a delusion of grandeur. So welcome! I hope you will be as pleased with the arrangement as I am. Poor fellow, this is surely a come-down from your former position.

Perhaps this is a penance—an expiation—an atonement you must make for filling so many pages of drama in your former existence with madmen.

Poor Shakespeare—it is certainly a reflection on your former genius to suggest that you must stalk with me over to "Three Building" because you are a maniac. And a still greater reflection on your taste and discrimination—if you had any choice in the matter—to think that you would come back to this world in this sort of a setting. But you did not choose me—I chose you—and you should not mind it—for here is an endless array of the theme you like best. And offering no disrespect to your very great genius—I am willing to wager that you will not find madness so intriguing when you have to be a mad person yourself—and have only those of your like to live with.

CHAPTER 2

THE DOCTOR WAS through again, just now. He is entirely too good looking. It is hard for a neurotic woman not to be sentimental about him—except that he is too damned wise. All these Doctors are. They have got us all analyzed and psychoanalyzed down to insignificant daubs of protoplasm—and personally, my Ego is not a bit flattered by the things they found out about it. Drat them! Life has settled into one burning obsession with me, to stir myself to the completion of their hypotheses—and convince them that if I am the exact duplicate of the twin sister of a Jack-Ass, then, they are most undeniably, very excellent—Veterinarians.

They call us insane—and in reality they are as inconsistent as we are, as flighty and changeable. This one in particular. One day he derides and ridicules me unmercifully; the next he talks to me sadly and this morning his eyes misted over with tears as he told me of the fate ahead. Damn him and all of his wisdom!

He has dinned into my ears a monotonous dirge—"Too Egotistical—too Egotistical—too Egotistical. Learn to think differently—Learn to think differently—Learn to think differently."— And how can I do it. How-how—can I do it? How the hell can I do it? I have tried to follow his suggestions but have not learned to think a bit differently. It was all wasted effort. Where has it got me?

Oh, he is a good Doctor alright. An excellent Doctor. All his conclusions are founded on excellent logic; the things he tells me are true—nauseatingly true. He is right, sickeningly right. In fact he is the very embodiment of all the virtue and wisdom in the world. For that reason, I detest him—passionately. But knowing these things does not keep me from the impulse to smack him down and that very impulse confirms the things he has told me.

I wish I could put a bell on him—so I would be aware when he starts probing around in the crooks and crannies of my crooked brain, hunting for phobias. He can do nothing with them when he finds them, so what is the use of hunting? Phobias are sensitive little critters—and it's like having a boil lanced, to have them probed into. He cannot cure them. All he does is go prowling around among them, knocking them over. When he finds an extra fine specimen he is as thrilled with his discovery as some be-spectacled bug-hunter who captures a rare type of beetle.

After he has found it, he does not know what to do with it. He cannot take it out and mount it or preserve it in alcohol. All he has in proof of his discovery is a long handled word to paste in his album. And I wish—Oh, how I wish, that I had the genius to take some of the smug self complacency out of him. He calls me Egotistical—and I am—but he suffers most bumptiously from it too. I do not see how he can fail to observe the symptoms in himself, when he can see them in others so clearly.

He stalks through here twice daily, in the pride of his lordly perfection. A great Modern Scientist inflated with wisdom, at work in his own laboratory. We who are patients here in the

"Hydro" are no longer people—merely things he has in test tubes. Experiments. Some of us are not successful. I, in particular, am an experiment of his that is no good at all and presently I shall be dumped over into "Three Building."

I know now how rats and rabbits and guinea pigs feel when they are vivisected. Vivisection is painful—and let those who think it isn't, get themselves pronounced insane—and get their brain analyzed by a modern psychologist.

The Doctor comes to you and in his most professional manner—softened down with such kindness as his mood at the time will permit, says you are too Egotistical and are going to wind up on "Three Building" unless you learn to think differently.

And if you really do have a bad case of infected, ingrowing Egotism—you get a pencil, the backs of old letters, sit down in the dormitory, call yourself Shakespeare and set out to tell all.

This is the Bug-house—the Bug-house—the Bug-house. Hooray for the Bug-house! It is also the Hydro—the Hydro—the Hydro. Hooray for the Hydro! The Bug-house is the place where Nuts are kept. The Hydro is the compartment where the very choice specimens are kept, watched, treated and worked on and done things to that have no more rhyme nor reason than a bath in flea soap has to a puppy. Perhaps it helps the pup—but he is not taken into the confidence of those who bathe him. He is just yanked up and plunged into the bath and never mind his protests. So are we. Never mind our protests. All that is done for us is good for us. It is just our hard luck that we have no comprehension. Yes—this is the Hydro—where is given all that is given to correct our abnormalities. And let me state that it is "Treatment"—and let me state that it is "Given."

The nurses are feeding one of the patients now. She would

/29/

not eat. Did not want to eat. But they are pouring the food down her anyway. They have a wooden peg in her mouth and are crouched behind a sheet held up like a shield, because the woman tries to sprew each mouthful upon them. She spits, howls, and curses simultaneously in one breath, she is tied down in a strait-jacket and can do nothing but spit and curse and howl. But how she is spitting and how she is cursing and how she is howling. Truly, it is a magnificent display of madness. Rage has mottled her face with a purple rash and the veins stand out on her neck from straining. Her mouth is open for cursing and one of the nurses reaches around the sheet with the feeding cup and splashes a great gulp of milk in her mouth. The other nurse catches her nose to shut off her breathing and covers her mouth with a towel. But she will not swallow and is strangling on the speech trapped in her throat. They gurgle up through the milk and curdle it but she will not swallow.

The sounds coming up through the milk cannot quite carry the shape of the curses; they lost their shape in the liquid, or else were gnashed into shapelessness by the grinding clench of her teeth. But, the spirit of them escapes through the milk and as they rise they make it gurgle and bubble and fly out in mist as though it were boiling. And she is mad enough to almost bring it to a boil without the aid of the curses. She hates herself for her inability to strangle to death before she must swallow. She is mad with her impotency and helplessness so she hates the nurses with fury unbelievable. Now they are finished and are leaving her, and her rage is directed at the whole world in general and spouts out against the Hydro ceiling in a scalding geyser of fury.

It is flung with such fury it does not seem possible a human voice can make such a noise and still retain the power to shape itself into speech. But it does—and even the force with which it hits the ceiling does not shatter the shape of the curses—for they are solid and substantial things and ride high above the tumult of the other noise she makes. They are constructed by Madness, out of double-strength, re-inforced hatred, and neither the force which expels them nor the crashing impact with the ceiling makes any dent in them.

You might think the awful oaths and profanities she releases with such disruptive explosion would be shattered to splinters on hitting the ceiling. But there is nothing anemic about these curses. They are large and full-bodied and bounding with vigor, and much more capable of denting the ceiling than the ceiling is of denting them, and when they hit it, their direction is changed. Instead of continuing their rocket flight upward, until they burned a hole through the stratosphere, the ceiling deflects them and they go bounding off against the walls, and roll back and forth in the aisles—so we are still getting the repeated impacts of the first ones, long after more violent ones have left her.

Never was there such a vocabulary! She could give a sailor lessons in the art of cursing. For her ability reaches far beyond Art. It is Genius!

She used to be a large woman, weighing more than two hundred pounds. Now she is shrunken to a fraction of that and her flesh hangs in loose folds about her tall frame. Her pelvic bones stick up like the rim of a bowl around her abdomen, which is a great mass of shrivelled wrinkles. She keeps it scratched and clawed and over-turned in great red welts and ridges. She has dug so deeply into her flesh she has turned it wrong side out in many places.

But I like "Claw-belly"—for she rose up and danced on the

day I was put into a jacket. She danced to my singing—a wild, whirling dance—and she was stark naked. She got tied down for her compliment to my singing. It was not beautiful singing— and I was stark mad or I would not have sung in the bug-house. And she was madder than I was, or she would not have danced to my singing. It was not beautiful dancing. You must be very beautiful indeed if you are able to get away with dancing without any clothes on and you must do it in the name of Art— and spell it with a very Capital A—or the police will interfere —or nurses will come with a strait-jacket.

There isn't the least bit of beauty in "Claw-belly's" carcass. So she got herself tied down; as did the "Camel," who danced too —but she did have the decency to drape her great hunched shoulders in a sheet, for, if possible, the "Camel" is uglier even than "Claw-belly." And because we were all stark mad and were all three tied down on neighboring beds, and because we each had to rave—(it is not possible to bear madness in silence)—we lay there and each fashioned songs to suit our own whims, and the Hydro was filled with more noise than usual.

The Doctor was so provoked at me he gave me two "Sick" Hypos, which make you so sick there is nothing at all in this world like them. Truly—if any one is hunting an experience that nothing in all this world is like, they should have a "Sick" hypo! For they produce a sickness that is past all imagining.

But that crazy clown in the strait-jacket wanted to sing—and I had to let her. If they had cut my head from my shoulders I could not have stopped her—even if death had been upon me, I could not have stopped her.

The Doctor thinks he has disposed of her nicely when he remembers the long-handled name for her. Ancient and primitive races said we were possessed of the devil—and I strongly suspect they were right. They had not reached the present day sophistication by inventing ten-syllable words for something they did not understand. So they called it the devil—and let it go at that.

Because my education has not progressed enough to give me comprehension of ten-syllable words—the painted symbol of some voodoo witch doctor would answer as well. But I will say this—the witch doctor does not live who could devise such an ingenuity as a sick-hypo to torture maniacs. Truly—it is a triumph in the ingenuities of modern medicine. I would rather eat bat-wings and mouse-ears—and whatever other ingredients might go into the preparations that witch doctors use in routing the devil—than to have my legs punctured with a sick-hypo.

Oh, there are other ingenious contrivances also used. They are all triumphs—and stand as great monuments to man's ingenuity. And they are used in a way which fulfills something an old poet said about "Man's inhumanity to man." One of the treatments is a "Pack." It is very simple. Also effective. You are simply—and securely—and unsnugly—tucked into a very wet bed—stark naked. And more water is added to make you still wetter—and enough more poured on to half drown you.

I am the only poor wretch who has been singled out for one since I have been here—so I do not know what they might do for another. At the time it was given me—I had not gone completely off the deep end and was not raving so I do not know what effect it would have had if I had been. Actual madness takes no thought at all for the condition of the body it is driving. It is an obsession too powerful in itself to take note of anything outside of itself.

Then there are drugs they give us, the mildest of which are "iprils." These small white tablets look like aspirin and do nothing but give you a terrible hang-over and headache the next day. There are sodium-amitols, a drug in a long green capsule which makes you as drunk as a sailor ashore. Also luminols, another drug which looks like an aspirin—and I had them, but I do not remember what they did to me nor how I felt afterwards, for I was too far gone in madness to have much concern for the things my body felt at the time.

Then there is paraldehyde—the magnificent! Paraldehyde has a flavor no single thing in this world is like. Paraldehyde, that triple strength, double distilled, concentrated essence of all the vile flavors in the universe. Someone has dubbed it "skunkoil"— but that name is only faintly suggestive, for no single word in the language is able to convey to another, all the revolting things a spoonful of it can release in your throat as you swallow. It has a rampant suggestiveness—and you recognize many full-bodied flavors of things so revolting in nature, the very thought of tasting them is nauseating.

It is a drug you drink—and if you refuse to take it, it is administered by the drenching method. Once you start to swallow —you do it in a hurry, or be asphyxiated on the spot. That is not exaggeration, either, it is so powerful you lose consciousness almost immediately. The flavor stays with you, long after all the other effects have worn off. I had a dose last Tuesday, I can still taste it and this is Saturday, I can roll my tongue against it, even as I write this.

They are giving the "Camel" a dose of it now—by the drenching method. She is choking and spluttering—and vows and swears she has been poisoned—and I do not wonder. If the flavor is any indication of its potency—one small dose could exterminate an army.

Then there are strait-jackets, and right here I want to pay my eternal tribute to a strait-jacket. Though it looks like an implement of torture designed in the Dark Ages, there are times when it looks like God's protecting arm round you. To feel yourself going berserk is a terrible sensation. When you feel all that is decent and right within you crumbling to ruins—and feel a creature emerging, of whom you know nothing except that she is about to possess herself of a massive and powerful body.

You feel her there awaiting and ready, crouched for the spring —and know that when your frail thong of self-control breaks you will be a maniac—raging, charging and bent on destruction. At such a time, a strait-jacket looks like God's angel sent to protect you. The very loveliest thing ever made.

CHAPTER 3

ANOTHER DAY HAS passed and Shakespeare is still out of a strait-jacket. Hurray for Shakespeare and for me, that I have the audacity to claim him. Poor Shakespeare, he may have been a genius in his former existence. In this one he is only a nut in a bug-house who must use his genius to keep out of a strait-jacket—and madness. And if he could pound the kinks out of his brain it would be as great a miracle as any genius could do. And because writing was his strong forte before, he has turned to it in his present predicament. Since I have the audacity to claim him he has a whole ream of hospital paper (he should not mind its having a hospital heading. If I had not claimed him, he would have had only the backs of such letters as come to me and a sheet of wrapping paper and what other scraps I could collect.

Patients who do not have Shakespeare as a delusion are allotted only two sheets of paper each Sunday to write their relatives).

But the pencil Shakespeare has is a scream. It is only the stub left after some nut finished dining. The eraser and the metal cap are gone, and the little bit left is chewed into splinters. It looks like something a pup had been gnawing. But it is not a puppy who has a belly full of splinters, it is one of the patients in here, for some of them have voracious appetites for inedibles.

This is the "hydro"—and the "hydro" is the mad-house in the mad-house. It is a mad-house—a bedlam—this instant. It is always in an uproar.

It is the basement of a wing at right angles with the rest of the building. Above are the wards where several hundred other patients are kept. They are placed in the various wards according to the system of grading, and are very far gone, indeed, if they fall into the "hydro." There are fourteen patients down here. All of them stark mad (except Shakespeare and I). The Doctor thinks we head the list. He will shortly oof us over onto "Three Building." That is even lower in this limbo than the "hydro." It is the sure-enough bottom.

But this is the "hydro"—hooray for the "hydro." It has a red cement floor, blue walls and a cream colored ceiling. There are twelve bright yellow beds stretching themselves at right angles to their reflections on the red floor. It makes a shrill pattern, blocked off in sharp angles of color. There are tall rows of grated windows on either side. A patient is standing at one of them now shrieking and trying to pick one of the padlocks holding the grates. She is so far gone in her madness she does not know she cannot pick a stout padlock with a safety-pin, but she jabs at it wildly. Nor does she know there are two other locks like the first one above her and out of her reach, and if she could get one of them picked with a safety pin the grates still would not open. Long before she could get all three picked, she would be tied down in a jacket. The nurses look in on us and check us every few minutes and write what we are doing on the charts which are our books of doom.

Those charts! One little check mark opposite some of the words printed on them, can just about seal our doom forever. They are big sheets of paper, held in metal frames. But the things on these sheets! Words—that could not be applicable anywhere except in an insane asylum. The words themselves are misleading—and have shocking, double meanings.

I had a great curiosity, while I was still up on the ward, to know some of the things written about us. For our fate hangs on the things in those charts. The reports are up to the nurses, and the Doctor bases his opinion and treatment on what they write about us.

One day when the nurses' backs were turned and the books of doom were unguarded, I availed myself of the chance to snoop through them—and was well repaid. I discovered among other things that I was marked "depressed and suicidal"—but I knew all about that. What I could not understand was how I had managed to escape some of the other classifications. For as I read them over, I thought surely some of them must fit me but there was no check opposite. I knew many of the things printed there could not possibly apply to me, but there was one caption which made me wonder. At the top of a list of unsavory suggestions was a small printed word "untidy." I thought I might miss the others but that one would catch me. I have never collected any medals for neatness or orderliness, which in my ignorance is what I thought the word meant. So I thought I had better begin to mend my disorderly, "untidy" ways. I re-arranged all my small personal belongings in a neat array the most persnickety old maid would not be ashamed of. I became a very model of neatness. I went around brushing small motes of dust, picking up ravelings—and kept myself carefully groomed for inspection.

More wasted effort. Not 'til I came to the "hydro" did I learn the meaning of the word "untidy." One of the patients just passed by with a dustpanful of human excreta the nurse made her clean up when one of the others evacuated all over the floor—as a cow does.

As she passed her face was filled with unutterable despair, and she held the unsavory load she carried at arm's length before her, turned her face backward and upward; and cried in a voice filled with anguish.

"O, my God—my God—I am so tired of cleaning out these Augean stables."

Words have strange meanings in an insane asylum—and Life flows on in strange channels. We live in a world apart. A Limbo of living dead. And it depends upon one's point of view, whether death is such a terrible thing. We are relieved of all responsible living—and nothing matters. We are so out of touch with the rest of the world the things happening on the great "Outside" might be happening on another planet.

We failed to meet the conditions of living—so the world dismissed us.

The patient who carried the dustpan has gone back to her picking and shrieking. Two others are raving their lungs out and a third one is dying. It is all a mad, scrambled confusion of sound and color and drama. There is no way to bring order out of such chaos—everything converges with something else— so that nothing can be traced to its source. Amid this setting, the mad drama of stark, naked, living continues—and Death stalks his prey slowly. He will not come quickly and free the fortunate one he has chosen from this tossing, seething delusion.

But Shakespeare liked madness—and maybe he can endure it. Were not some of his most dramatic characters mad-men? Did he not fill many pages about them? If I could have just a little bit of his seeing perhaps I might change my own viewpoint a little. Poor Shakespeare—it is a cruel expiation. In one life-time, a genius; in the next one—a blacksmith. A blacksmith; who must pound his brain straight on an anvil of hospital paper—with a hammer that is only the stub of a pencil left behind when some nut finished dining.

Bah! Shakespeare—you've got things in a worse mess than they were. Here I caught on to you and you try to run out on me already. You think you can't stand it. And you were the guy who used to write about madness. So—. It was only drama which was written and not real. Well, my dear Shakespeare, here it is before you and it is real. No one in the world could catch the real significance and meaning of life in the "Hydro." If you could catch it—no one in the world could understand it. So go on and play marbles—and spin stories of fiction—and choose characters who live life lightly—for Madness is a subject for only God and the Doctors to deal with.

That is why your previous writings were so highly appreciated by a world that did not have the courage to do its own seeing. Because we are all part of life, we cannot look at it nakedly, with straight-forward seeing. So we pay great prices to those who will see it and tell about it in pleasant words. We are spared the pain of learning what it all means. And to get right back at you, Shakespeare, if you stick around the "hydro," you will learn the meaning of madness by grim first hand experience. Then, if you are able to write of it as glibly as you did when you spun it of fancy—you will indeed be a genius—or a jackass.

After this you will turn a deaf ear to any nut in an insane asylum who tries to choose you as a delusion of grandeur. Here-after—forever—you will come only to someone who wants to write about the birds and the bees and the flowers that bloom in the spring, tra-la. For you will have washed your hands of madness forever.

The "hydro" is an eddying backwash where odd pieces of flotsam are carried deeper and deeper to emerge again in "Three Building"—there to sink from sight forever. There is nowhere in the world another place like it—except perhaps, some other "hydro" in some other insane asylum. Sometimes there are more patients than there are beds. Starched nurses bring them each morning and come to take them back to the wards each evening.

Those who have charge of the traffic are often hard put to make disposition of the vast cargo of human derelicts the tide of life brings to the mad-house. Unless the world can discover how to stop the flood at its source, it must rise to wonder how small a remnant will be left, when the influx into madness is ended. They pour into this institution faster than the State can assemble equipment to house them.

Among all the hundreds of patients in this institution is enough material to build "awful warnings" for the whole race.

At the head of the list is a middle-aged woman of stern virginal purity. I suppose she is still a virgin, but the sternness has grown and developed into something grim and terrible; and the "purity" has been replaced by a maniacal obscenity which is revolting.

Now, in the middle years of her life she has left behind both natural modesty and her exalted idea of purity; since madness has claimed her—she has been swept far into unspeakable lewdness. She is so far gone into madness that she fashioned a set of male genitals out of a snuff box. She stands naked before all who may see her and gives voice to her madness by shrieking such foulness the very air around her is crawling and stinking with it. Until others who are mad also, and not easily shocked by such exhibitions, cannot endure the sight of her—who at one time in her life was modest to a point of prudery.

Prudery, "what crimes are committed in thy name." Here she

stands, unashamed, uninhibited—in fact completely oblivious to those around her. A set, concentrated look of impotent passion wreathes her eyes. Her lips are opened—mouthing her obscenities. Her hands rending and tearing already torn flesh. And she came here a virgin. But wait, did she come here because she was a virgin? Or did she come here because some other circumstance forced it?

I do not know what the reason back of such disintegration is. She has lived up to the code of her life, both former and latter, with all the power of her being. And if one extreme does follow another—then she is indeed a terrible warning to all who may see her. A warning not to get so exalted in righteousness—lest the thing which is their life should rebel and show the extent of its power in retaliation for being controlled too severely.

She was so sure of her perfection that she denied the very existence of impulses she counted evil. Or else she felt so much responsibility for them that now she has passed the stage of responsibility altogether. Now she is no more responsible for her acts than the typhoon that rages—she is completely demented.

And I, who am no part of a preacher, think I see a meaning in what the Great Teacher meant when he warned those whom he taught "Not to cast their pearls before swine, lest they trample them, and turn again and rend them."

Now, all that is decent and right within her is trampled under the feet of her madness—and her very life will be soon trampled out in the general destruction—for she will most likely die in her raving.

Bestials, sadists, homo-sexuals and those poor miserable persons who are what is politely termed "over-sexed" do not often land here. Those are things peculiar to the great civilized world.

Those people seek and find their relief in and amongst their own kind. The mere fact they do find the necessary outlet prevents, or at least delays, their confinement.

Those who, through some peculiar quirk find such things necessary or desirable, find them in the civilized world. And in the finding they automatically preclude the possibilities, or at least the probabilities, of arriving here.

This is no treatise on the subject, I hold no brief for such things. We who are demented only set forth these facts in defense of ourselves against the whispered charges of Mr. and Mrs. Grundy.

We are here because we couldn't take it, whatever it was. In the main, we are not here because we were oversexed or perverted or sadistic, no—we are here because we are just plain crazy. Because we had mothers or fathers or even grandparents who should not have been allowed the "privilege of procreation." We are here because of such little things as the "power of suggestion." We are here because we listened to and believed all those things we saw and felt as a danger.

The homo-sexual simply finds another of the same ilk. The pervert finds someone in perversion. The sadist finds someone who, too, is sadistic—and they do not show up here. They are "civilized."

And then, oh yes, then we, the demented, must stand by and see our moralizing, our self-righteous, we-don't-do-it, attitude knocked into a cocked hat by the exhibition we have just witnessed. We will witness it again—and again, because here is the exception which proves the rule. Tomorrow or maybe even tonight will come one of those incommunicable messages, one to the other and someone—perhaps the Pagan, perhaps "Clawbelly," maybe even the Camel will receive some indefinable message and—if they are not in a strait-jacket, answer the primeval urge. Unknowingly and involuntarily, as an animal does. Physical hungers, whether for food, drink or anything else is automatic, and in here, without the veneer of civilization as protector --- automatically answered, unless the nurses intervene.

We hear of visitors frightened by the bestial appearance of the inmates. The nurses recount these things in glee. A man and his wife, for instance, passing this place plan to stroll through on a visit to satisfy their morbid curiosity. They'll be cautioned by the attendants to remain close together. They would do this anyway. Then they'll go home and recount with delicious chills how the male patients looked at the women. How they shouted ribald remarks. They might even add a few embellishments to show they were followed about or of some attempted attack.

Most of it will be pure fiction, unless the appearance of the visitors coincides with some part of the inmate's delusion at that very moment, the visitors will be looked at—but never seen. My friend, Shakespeare, and I will remember that even he could never imagine all the bits of fiction scattered by casual visitors. And life will go on in the Hydro.

So much for my analyzing—and what do I know about it? Nothing, exactly nothing. And yet I know everything, I have been through it. There is no teacher so convincing as experience, but experience does not equip the student she teaches with a technical vocabulary of ten-syllable words. Once you have left it, and seen the very force of yourself flow out in a stream of insanity you get a pencil and sit down and write; anything —anything to try and forestall a repetition of your experience.

There is even a method in the madness of calling yourself Shakespeare. Since Shakespeare and I have kept ourselves out of a strait-jacket for nearly a week, those who have the care of us can think what they like of our methods. They could give us no suggestions of how to do the impossible. They said it was an impossibility for anyone as insane as I was—before Shakespeare came to me—to cope with the problem.

Before that, they insisted there was nothing at all wrong with my head because I could answer all the stupid questions they asked me. There are many patients here who have an I.Q. higher than some still on the "outside." A person may have an I.Q. high enough to be well above average—and still not be able to apply it, to cope with some problem that cannot be coped with. They give me a pain—with their exalted idea of the two-by-four wisdom they think is so inclusive; for when it comes to a show-down, it is not inclusive enough to offer a solution to any problem of life.

They have endless formulas which may be very informative to them—but they can give little information to those whom they are trying to deliver from madness. It all boils down to this—if we who are entangled in madness are to be delivered, we must deliver ourselves—they cannot help us. I do not resent the fact they are unable to help us. I do resent the fact they take such pride to themselves for wisdom they do not possess.

They probe around, and drag this out and look at it—and that out, and look at it. You submit with what grace you have—and cooperate with what intelligence you have. Finally they emerge with a very solemn face and deliver a solemn pronouncement, (a fact you have known all your life), "You are too Egotistical."

One day a great Doctor who was very wise;
Fell down in a fit—and near died of surprise
When a germ he was trying to analyze

Looked up through the lens and winked in his eyes
And said, plain as day—in a microbe-like way
"I know you're a Doctor the world views with pride
While I'm little of nothing that's been classified;
But I really admire the way you have tried
And I'd offer my help, if I thought you'd divide
And play fair with the pay that will come your way
When the laws of my being you fully decide."

Oh, my goodness me—I am in the same class
As the microbe who dared squint up through the glass
And address a great scientist with so much "brass."
The metaphor's clumsy—the truth is—Alas,
I'm transparent as air; in fact nothing there
He's unravelled me down to the bare protoplasm
With a flick of the wrist—there was nothing to
fathom.
Plumbed the depth of my soul—not much of a chasm;
Stripped my poor Ego bare—left it shivering there.
God tempers the breeze to the lambs that are shorn
But He leaves me to freeze—more nude than when
born.

Yes; we who are here are much less interesting than so many
germs in test tubes. But it strikes me that even things in test
tubes might be most damned important to themselves. I can
speak for them, because I am one of them—and I do not in the
least mind admitting that I am important to Me. Whether or not
my life is of any importance to any other creature in the world
—it is to me.

I will even go further. Regardless of what others may think
of me or of what worth I may or may not be to the general
scheme of things; there is no use denying that, to myself at
least, I am the most interesting specimen of God's creativeness

in existence. And Life; even in a test tube, is a momentous experience. Even if the life we live in the Hydro is a worm's life—we worms are alive and squirming.

Down one side of our worm-hive in the room where the worms' beds are, politely called the dormitory—are four huge bathtubs—almost as big and tall as the beds. They were designed for hydro-therapy, the patient to be suspended on a hammock in the water. But the water here is sandy and gritty and could not be used in the delicate mechanism. So, all the rods and knobs and wheels and gadgets on the outside of the tub are of value only as something to polish. That is a help—for anything on which time can be consumed in an insane asylum is to be caught at and used to the last minute possible.

But, if the bath-tubs cannot be used for the purpose for which they were designed, at least they are the last word in luxury to bathe in. They approach the old Roman ideal of plenty of water. When they are well-filled a worm as long as I am; and I crowd six feet, can float in them touching no part of the porcelain. In fact, I was doing just that yesterday, when a little relief nurse came tearing back, pulled the stopper and carried it away with her. Because I am marked "suicidal" she thought I was trying to drown myself—at least that's what she told me. I tried to convince her I had no designs on my life, but she would not believe me, would not stay to hear me, but took the stopper to lock up with the ice-pick and paring knife. The stoppers are heavy rounds of metal and are kept out of sight along with everything else that might possibly suggest a weapon. For that same reason, we are not even allowed a nail-file. When our nails need trimming, the nurses trim them so closely they cannot be used to fight with. They trim them almost into the quick; not letting the scissors out of their hands.

There is another room called the day hall. On one side are chairs. On the other is a table, ice-box and cabinet of heavy home-woodshop construction. A short hall goes from the day hall to the "hydro" door. On one side is the stool-room, which has four stools at one side and a kitchen sink at the other. The flush-boxes are built into the walls so the plumbing may not be tampered with. For the same reason the radiators are all suspended a few inches from the ceiling.

One of the patients washes in the stools because she thinks the water in the tap has lye in it. And there are many people in the world who would squirm at the idea of using the stools for the purpose for which they were designed, because there are some terrible diseases down here. The nurses have a picture-frame which they use as an auxiliary seat.

Across the hall from the stool-room is the linen room. The private sanctum-sanctorum of the nurses. It is only a cubbyhole but they spend their time, between checking and watching us, in there.

Next to the linen room is the "side-room." It is only a cubbyhole, too. Just large enough to hold a person who must be shut away with their madness in solitary confinement. There is nothing in it except a bed. We take turns occupying it, the preference falling to the one who is raving the loudest.

CHAPTER 4

PEOPLE WHO LIVE in the "hydro" have the power to create worlds out of delusion. Worlds as different from the world of ordinary living as a citizen on the "outside" could imagine in his wildest moments of fancy. Here everything is in a topsy-turvey condition and nothing looks right or familiar. It differs as greatly as would be the difference in finding yourself in a world where people stood on their heads and walked on the ceiling and went backwards in order to read something before them. There is nothing inconsistent to any of us in the pursuit of our strange fancies; even though we may be shocked at the strange things we see in the others.

We call each other crazy and are all in the same boat together. So if I want to call myself Shakespeare, and write of the others, I only follow the good old custom of mania in choosing a patron as a delusion of grandeur. We cannot cope with life as we find it, nor can we escape it or adjust ourselves to it. So we are given the power to create some sort of world we can deal with. The worlds created are as varied as there are minds to create them. Each one is strictly private and cannot be shared by another. It is much more real than reality. For nothing that happens to a sane mortal in the common-place world of ordinary living, can approach the startling intensity of things going on in delusion. There is a sharpness—a shrillness—a piercing intensity which thrusts itself through the consciousness and is so much more convincing than the blunt edge of reason, that even if the two are conflicting there is no choice between them. Reason is beaten, dismissed and defeated at the very outset, it cannot contend with the saber edge of delusion.

I shall have to whet my eyes to sharper seeing than I have at present if I am to see much deeper than the fantastic exteriors their odd souls are wrapped in. For I do not understand them, I do not understand myself—and I am one of them.

"Claw-belly," for instance. What an odd creature she is, lying there, howling and singing and spitting and cursing. The nurse is pinning a sheet into a tent over the head of her bed now to force her to use her spittle for home consumption. Presently the inside of the tent will be dripping with it.

And the Skeleton—who is running back and forth down the aisle and past the windows as an animal paces its cage. Now she is standing on tip-toe and the shrieks coming from her almost lift the ceiling. She is the most fleshless creature imaginable.

There is not enough muscle and tissue padding her bones to conceal their outline. She is only a skeleton with a moth-eaten blanket of skin thrown around it. And mad, stark, stark mad. Howling and shrieking and tearing at the loose folds of skin about her.

The Camel, whose canvas strait-jacket is rising and falling like a great bellows, from her heavy breathing in sleep, induced by paraldehyde. She is kept drugged most of the time—for she does love to rave—and is such a sociable soul she wants to share everything with another.

She has such an odd slant on things and such a ludicrous humor, that to be able to catch her view-point is to be convulsed into hysterics. She is a big woman, of ungainly proportions. Her shoulders bulge outward in a great curving hump like a camel's; and a similarity is further noticeable in her loose, angling gait when she walks. That is, when she gets a chance to walk, since she is kept in a jacket and drugged most of the time.

The Medicine-maker. I call her that because on the day I was brought to the "hydro" she was sitting out in the day hall, with a heavy over-hanging black forelock brought down from her forehead and tied with a strip of bath-toweling. She sprang out before me, holding the fantastic adornment in a dramatic and meaningful gesture—then flung her arms wide and bowed low before me in welcome. She straightened, then folded her arms on her chest and looked at me. Her piercing black eyes behind the barricade of the barbarous symbol, glittered brightly with madness.

She so transfixed me with the power of suggestion that what she said to me seemed very convincing:

"Welcome, stranger—welcome among us. But, remember, remember always that I am the great Medicine-maker of this tribe."

But the Chieftains who are higher in power than she is have kept her tied down in a jacket for many long weeks. She lies there in silence and hatred. The thoughts filling her brain are known to no one. There is a black pall of madness; brooding, waiting—and watching. It emanates from her and settles around her in sinister foreboding silence.

To feel her eyes sweep you is to feel a chillness blown from caverns of hatred, black, vast and bottomless. To meet her eyes squarely is to feel something within you turn away quickly, chilled with the knowledge that it has seen naked madness— heavy, and pregnant with horror unborn.

Even though she is tied down and helpless—there is something about her which generates fear in all others. And the Doctors and nurses are cautious as they deal with her.

There is the Opera singer—a small, pitiful figure of a woman whose life is an endless tragedy—and whose only escape from the pressure of pain is to slip out into madness, and find relief in her delusion that she is a great opera singer. She is like nothing in the world so much as a little brown field mouse. A little brown field mouse in a trap. She it is who washes in the stools because she thinks there is lye in the tap water. She fears the harshness of lye will disfigure the loveliness that has triumphantly sung before kings.

Then the Pagan; as beautiful and graceful a creature as ever stalked through a "hydro" stark naked. Clothes are an encumbrance she has dispensed with forever—if she has her way. The nurses tie something around her or shut her up in the stool-room about the time they expect the Doctor on his rounds. But other than that she can go as she likes—and she likes to go naked.

She will stand and sing at a window in the feminine of whatever kind of a voice Cab Calloway has, and end her song by shrieking. Cry—after cry—after cry. The naked and uncheckable out-pourings of her own soul. There is nothing else in the universe like them.

To see such a creature as she is stand naked—and howling with madness, is to wonder whether or not she is real; or an illusion both grim and lovely. It does not seem possible life could be such a grim sculptor as to carve from smooth, living beauty the exquisite details of a cameo, then set such lovely perfection in a mounting of madness. Yet—there she is. A beautiful creature. And I know she is real for illusions produce ideas only, not matter. It was from her that the dust-pan of pollution was carried.

Then there is the Farm-woman, lying on her bed with her head covered, fighting an ever-losing battle with longing. Longing so intense, that in itself it is madness. Longing of so fierce a nature it has the power to turn her into a maniac. A life-time filled with fierce wanting.

The thing she longs for, such a small thing it does not seem right that life could be cruel enough to deny it. When there is a world full of wilderness and uncultivation—she cannot have a small over-turned corner in which she can make a garden.

There is also the Student, sitting with her feet sprawled in an ungainly posture, because whoever seated her did not take the trouble to arrange her limbs in a graceful, or even comfortable position. She will sit as she was seated, until someone comes and moves her. She has no more motivation or seeming consciousness of life than a French doll.

She used to be a brilliant student in her years of schooling and would still be in the class-room if this thing had not overtaken her. She is not so devoid of feeling as her conduct indicates.

One time when the nurse dragged her along to the library for exercise, she was amazed to see the girl stand and gaze, as one transfixed, upon the shelves of books before her. Whereas before, she had been so indifferent those who saw her wondered whether she had any consciousness at all. The books she looked at not only aroused interest but interest of so poignant and painful a nature as to awaken tears.

She stood before the book-case and all within her was expended in a flood of weeping. No teasing, tenderness or coaxing could induce her to take a book into her hand. No amount of persuasion drew her an explanation of why she wept. The tears were her own secret soul's expression of some pain known only to itself—nor did she impart the reason or seek for understanding in any other. Now she is taken often to the library in the hopes she will produce the phenomenon of tears again.

There is the Dancer, a young mother, who before the days of motherhood earned a degree in college. Now, she is so far gone in madness they brought her to the "hydro" when they found her standing at one of the windows on the ward upstairs, broadcasting a radio message to the President through a hand-mirror. She has many odd delusions and insists she is one of the officials, and the sweetheart of one of the Doctors; and each of them have too much dignity to be flattered. She is a pretty girl—her one flaw in looks is a missing front tooth, the result of "pegging".

Then there is the Tragedy. She it is whom Death has laid his hand on—yet will not pluck quickly lest there be a few dregs undrained in the bottom of the grim cup of madness. She dies a death too horrible for thinking, nor does she know she is dying—but has livid knowledge only of the madness which burned her life to an ember.

Her mother went this way before her, in this same institution. This daughter, not yet twenty; cannot follow till she has paid with the last ounce of quivering life within her for her folly. The folly of choosing for a mother a syphilitic woman. And there is a younger sister over whom is hanging the dread of penalty of "the sins of the father."

Because the judgment of unborn babies is notoriously poor judgment—some day the State will have the courage to say who shall appoint themselves to the office of parenthood.

The nurses are coming now to feed her—from the opposite end of the intestinal tract through which food is usually received into the body. She does not know they feed her, or that she is

/56/

dying. Yet there is no hope for her and the end is only a matter of waiting.

The next I call the Mother. I am sitting at the foot of the bed to which she is tied. She hates her jacket so much she cannot endure it. She has been pleading with me to untie her and has exhausted her almost inexhaustible supply of unsavory labels for me because I wouldn't. Now she is calling in a sing-song voice for some "Blue Jacket Boys" to come and untie her. She goes on at length to tell them of the indignities heaped upon her. She is struggling with every breath to release herself—for she cannot bear the restraint of being tied.

Now she has scooted down until she is about to choke herself against the stout bedticking straps crossed under her chin. Her face is very red and the veins stand out on her forehead from the strain. The straps bind across her wind-pipe so she can hardly breathe but her speech continues in muffled gasps. Oh, she has nearly wiggled out! I believe she will make it! She will have to hurry as the nurses are almost through with the sick patient. She is going to make it, I do believe. If she can force her head through the opening in the straps she will. One more grunt, one more strain, one more great wrenching effort will do it.

She did it! She did it! Her arms are wiggling frantically against the ties, the straps cut into the soft flesh of her shoulder and the skin is red from friction. But the nurses are coming. They have caught her and are untying the knots and straps she is tangled in.

She is happy, she thinks they are releasing her. But they are not. They only untied the knots to tie her back again tighter than ever. Now she knows what they do and is shrieking to them and pleading to be allowed to go.

"Don't do that, please don't do that!! Oh, you Bitch." "Let me alone, let me alone,—you,—you." More profanity—and now she is shrieking to one of her children, "Jerry—Jerry—Grab that Knife and Come in Here and Kill These People."

Now it is finished, she is tied so tightly she can hardly breathe; and because she was so nearly out but couldn't quite make it, she is in despair and sobbing like a child:

"I can't stand it, I can't stand it"—first, piteously.

"I can't stand it, I can't stand it"—then entreatingly.

"I can't stand it, I can't stand it"—and again, louder, demandingly. Finally a raging shriek at the top of her lungs.

"I Can't Stand it! I Can't Stand it!"

Claw-belly's voice rolled out from under her tent, soaked with the moisture of her dripping spittle. "O God, O God, O God, O God!!! If she can't stand it, O God, let her set it down, O God, or let her hang it on a nail, O God, or anything, O God, but make her shut up, O God."

Claw-belly is in a very religious mood but I doubt if there is very much reverence in it. She is singing "Jesus, Lover of My Soul." Another patient is joining in, a third follows. They all sing in a different key and tempo. The result is fearful and wonderful but not very tuneful. If the Camel was awake she would join them, too, and then the harmony would really be gummed up. She has a voice like a steam caliope, but the way she drags it out so long makes you think the keys are stuck. This is bad enough without her contribution to the general inharmony. One of them is midway in the second verse and the other is on the last line of the chorus.

Claw-belly has given it up altogether and is fitting the tune to a stream of profanities that are very odd words to sing to sacred music. Now she is chanting in a very good contralto, words, words, meaningless words of her own invention and

/58/

coinage but of constantly repeated rhyme and rhythm. Oh, I have it now. She is taking every profane word in her vocabulary and is going through the whole alphabet to create new words that rhyme with each one she chose as a pattern. So that is how she developed such a genius for profanity!!

The Skeleton is running back and forth before the windows shrieking and howling. I wonder she has not rubbed the few remaining ounces of flesh from her chattering bones by her frantic wringing and gripping and clutching. Now she is literally tearing at the flesh of her shoulders. She is actually frothing at the mouth and it overflows faster than she can think to turn and spit into one of the bathtubs.

She ran a few steps toward the door and then turned back to the window with a still wilder shriek to a man she saw passing. She frantically offers him six hundred dollars if he will come open her window. She makes two very distinct syllables of the word "window" and the accent is a shriek that falls on the "dow."

Now she is spitting again but does not bother to aim it into the bathtub. It falls where gravity guides it. Her gown is ripped open from neck to hem and the protruding bulge of her abdomen catches the drooling spittle as it flows in streams to the floor. She is not an appetizing sight to look upon. Now it is streaming down faster from her mouth, which is open and straining with horror as shriek after shriek comes from her throat and her eyes are glued in my direction.

But she sees nothing, she feels only some terror stalking her. Her eyes do not look like human eyes. Even the shape of them is changed by the terror of the things she sees. Now she is coming toward me. Her shrieks beat against my ears. Shrieks that stream out from the same source which sets her mouth drooling.

What can I do to help her? Nothing, exactly nothing. I cannot help her and I cannot hide my eyes from seeing her. It is better not to know there are such things as she feels in the world than to see what she suffers and be unable to help her.

But since she feels as she does, I am glad she can let a little of the pressure out by howling and tearing at her flesh. The things she feels cannot be borne in silence; and although what she is doing is senseless, it is better for her to give expression to it in howls and clutchings than to try to restrain it altogether.

She would give me the jitters if there was anything left in me to jitter. So go to it, old rattling bones, Howl—and more power to your howling! Yell it out, and maybe when you get through you will find a pencil that some nut chewed up and sit down and write about me. I may be howling next, you never can tell. Only I do not feel like it now. The example you are setting is not a temptation, just an awful warning.

It is meal-time again. It does not differ greatly from feeding time in a zoo. The uproar with Claw-belly is on again, and it is an exact repetition of the other occasion and the next meal will be the same and the next and the next. The Medicine-maker will not eat, either, but they let her alone for days at a time, and she lies there in hatred and silence. The little brown Field-mouse is hiding green onions under her pillow.

The beautiful naked Pagan has appropriated two trays and has stacked as much bread as would make an ordinary loaf on one of them and an extra cup of milk on the other. She is darting past, her naked legs flying as she runs to her bed with the Farm-woman after her. The Farm-woman has charge of the serving-table, but no matter what she is doing she always keeps one eye on the Pagan who has such a voracious appetite that she eats as much at one meal as six lumber-jacks would eat in one day. Her method of doing it is very simple. She will eat all she can hold,

eat till her stomach is far distended, then take time out for dis-
gorging to increase her capacity. Then she will dart up to the serving table and plunge her hands into what ever bucket of food is
nearest.

One of the nurses gave Bones a tray and told her to feed one
of the others. She shrieked when she took it and said she could
not do it. But she is doing it in a truly original manner. She is so
filled with despair she is taking no notice of what she is doing.
The patient she is feeding is hungry, her mouth is open very
wide to try to catch all the food being spilled in her hair and on
her pillow.

There is a green onion on her tray, and Bones saw her mouth
gaping and picked up the onion, thrusting it end-ways all the
way down her throat. Without waiting for her to get it up into
her teeth so she could chew it, she picked up a whole frankfurter
and thrust it in with the onion. Then she tamped both in with
a whole slice of bread so the one who is tied can neither chew,
swallow nor speak and it stretching and straining her neck like
a goose choked on corn. And Bones is cramming more bread in
her mouth.

Well, she did it! I would have sworn it was impossible but she
twisted and squirmed and stretched her neck longer and swallowed and believe it or not, Mr. Ripley, her mouth is gaping and
empty.

The Pagan and the Farm-woman are in the midst of another
conflict. The Farm-woman caught her hands as they flashed into
a bucket and wrenched them aside, then over head and the
Pagan stands there panting with eagerness as she looks at the
buckets.

"All of it, all of it, oh, let me have all of it."

Her mouth is drooling and her eyes are dilated with great

longing. Now she is really fighting to get what she wants. She cannot possibly be hungry, she has had two trays already with another serving or two of almost everything. What could make her feel that way towards frankfurters and beans, I can't imagine.

The food is not so bad there need be a great complaint made about it, but neither is it good enough to excite such craving as that. She is positively bulging already. But she got a third tray and is going back to her bed content. Food, and no raiment, seems to make Pagan happy.

The food is prepared in the general kitchen and at meal time one or two of the patients go with a nurse to get it. It is served by the nurses and the Farm-woman on aluminum plates, ridged and divided; our only silver is spoons, knives and forks being possible weapons. The cups are of aluminum. For the patients who will not eat there are feeding cups and the "peg." The feeding cups are like granite teapots with the spout at one side.

At one time when one of the patients was determined not to eat and enraged that they fed her, she gnashed her teeth through the peg and broke off some of the porcelain. The peg has been gnashed against so much the stout oak is prickly with splinters. The bleaching of many washings cannot quite hide its smoky look from being so often exposed to sulphurous curses.

There is the "Madam." That name really fits her. The day she was brought in was really a red letter one in the "hydro."

She had scarcely settled down on a bed when she began to "organize the girls." Then she looked about for the linen supply closets.

Going over to "Claw-belly," she looked at her disapprovingly and sniffed, "Humph, you'll never get any business, guess we better get rid of you right now. Go on over to Captain Charlie's. He'll send you down to New Orleans. That's the only place you're fit to work."

After she had examined us all critically and, I must add, disappointedly, she remarked, "Looks like I'm really stuck with sumpin' this time. How in hell can I be expected to make this place pay off? Grated windows are okay to keep the girls in, but those damn bars on the door will keep the cash customers out. Sumpin's gotta be done. Where the hell is the porter? Get 'im down here right now. Tell 'im to get those damn doors mounted on two-way hinges."

Then she turned, startled by the clammy fingers of the woman who had made the snuff box instrument.

Clutching the "Madam" in a fierce grip she pled, excitedly, "Can I be your helper? Can I? I want to be your right hand man whenever you get started. I want to be the door man and see "men" come in. I want to see them as they pick and choose the girls. One of 'em might pick me. Wouldn't that be swell?"

The "Madam" turned to her and said, venomously, "Get the hell away from me, you old bag. Who do you think would come in this damn house if you were on the door? Go on, beat it before I send you down to New Orleans with that other old beat up bag-of-bones. A man wouldn't even pay you a quarter. Scram!"

Old Snuffy went away mumbling to herself. "Here I am, a respectable, upstanding member of the Bridge Club and she won't even let me be the door man. I'll fix her. I'll get me a place of my own. That's what I'll do. I'll get a place and I won't let her get near it. If she comes around and bothers me I'll have the mayor take her license away. That's what I'll do.

"I'll tell him she's got syphilis and gonorrhea and chancres on her lips. I'll tell him she's even got cancers on her breasts, 'n pockmarks on her belly and that she takes a douche with battery acid. I'll fix her. I'll tell 'im she wears a girdle to hold her "behind" down, an uplift to hold her breasts up but she don't need a skull cap to hold her brains in. The old bitch. That'll make 'er wish she'da let me be the doorman 'n watch the men. I wanta see the men, dammit, somebody get me a man quick. They took my snuff box away and I gotta have a man."

While the "Madam" was busily, and happily, making her plans to "do business," she strolled past me. When she saw the huge bulk of me she yelled,

"My God, what have I got into? You big ox, what the hell do you think you're doing in here? Who asked you to 'work' here? Jeez, how can I get started with such girls? Whereinells the good lookers? Who are the 'come ons' for this joint, anyhow? Gotta do some advertising of some kind. Can't set here on my can and do any good with this bunch. Jesus H. Christ, go way —you look like you're crazy!"

The last remark made me very angry. I didn't think I looked any more crazy than she did so I exclaimed: "I'm crazy! you're crazy! The whole bunch are crazy! Come down off your high-horse and cut out the fancy plans. You aren't going to start any 'place.' Neither is Snuffy. You are both going to shut up and settle down. Quit interfering with me. Can't you see I'm busy. Shakespeare and I are bringing Hamlet up to date. Get away, you—you Banquo's Ghost, go be a death's head somewhere else."

Not daunted in the least, "Madam" continued her tour of inspection.

Meeting the Pagan, who was just coming out of the stool room; although I don't know why; she never used them, the Madam gasped, "My God, I was wrong. Here's what I need, she's beautiful, whatta face, whatta figure. Hold still a minute Dearie, I wanta see you better, straighten up your shoulders so's your breasts 'ill stick out, and you'll drive 'em crazy. You and me are gonna do some business. How much can you handle. Jeez, we'll get twenty-bucks a throw, and twenty-five throws a day or my name ain't Sioux City Sue. Jeez, I'll get me a coupla gals from Paris to do the 'fancy flips' 'n you c'n be the 'straight girl'. We'll clean up. We'll make so damn much money they'll have us in Alcatraz with old Al Capone, fer evadin' the income tax. Whatta racket, whatta racket. Let them damn bureau of 'infernal revenuers' come on. They won't catch me. We'll hide the money in our brassieres and if they do start to search fer it they'll fergit what they're lookin' fer!"

The Pagan only stood there, placidly, contentedly, and did what she should have done in the stool room. Only God knows why they don't keep a diaper on her, even if they have to chain it.

Months later, the Madam, who, behind her bloated, puffy appearance still bore traces of a delicate beauty told me:

"I got a daughter, see, a beautiful girl. Very nice, too, or at least she was. I had sent her to a boarding school in the East. Kept her there so she wouldn't know how I made my money, see. I was proud of her and had all kinds o' plans so's she wouldn't ever find out about me. Was gonna quit and tell her her daddy was dead and had left me a lotta dough, see."

"All of a sudden she quit writin' to me and I got frantic. Had the dicks throw out a drag, see. But no luck, Geneva had just disappeared and I nearly went nuts."

"I was just about ready to close up and go look for her when I decided that was silly. I'd just let Edna take over while I went to New York to start a search."

"I was gone several months. No luck, nary a trace of my daughter. Then I sorta gave up and decided maybe she'd heard about me and didn't wanta know me any more. So I came back to the 'house.' It was a 'nice' place then. All fancy drapes 'n such. Private rooms with 'high yeller' maids, who didn't always stop at bein' maids. They managed to pick up quite a few bucks on the side. Fact is, they could sometimes get more than the other gals from certain fellows."

"There was a Fiji islander a pearl trader brought me once when I was in San Francisco who; but never mind, I'll tell you about her some other time. I was telling you about comin' home and startin' to check up with Edna."

"She dumped a basket full of greenbacks in my lap and started in to tell me about a new girl she'd taken on. Said she had coal black hair, a figger like a statue and a face like an angel."

"Edna rambled on, tellin' me how the gal had every customer crazy about her. She did things to them none o' the other girls, even the 'yellers' could think of, 'n then told me how she was a never-get-enough sort of a girl. She could handle men as fast as she could sorta clean up and never seemed to get tired. Told me she often cracked that old joke about having to quit 'cause her feet were getting tired."

"Not thinking much about it, while my mind was still on Geneva, I started on upstairs when I got the idea of looking in on this new Cleopatra."

"She wasn't busy when I knocked so she said sweetly, 'Come in.' I opened the door and walked in. There she sat over in a dim corner of the room, brushing her long black hair."

"I walked over toward her as she turned around and said, 'Hello Mamma, I'm glad you're back. Now maybe we can do some real business in this two-bit, jerk-water joint.'"

As she said this the "Madam" began to pace back and forth nervously; a troubled expression on her face was superseded by venom and she began to scream. "Get me the Mayor. Get the Chief of Police. Get the Governor. I gotta get outta here. What the hell you think I been payin' for. Get those bastards on the phone- tell 'em they better spring me quick or I'll talk, I'll yell, I'll scream. I'll make 'em wish they'd never taken my money. Get me the reporters. I wanta tell 'em something. I wanta give 'em a story that'll blow the lid off. 'Spose they have got a campaign on. Tell 'em to get me outa here 'fore I lose 'em an election. Think they c'n doublecross me, do they, I'll show 'em. You tell those dirty skunks if they don't bail me out by sundown I'm gonna talk, see. And when I talk I got sumpin' to say. Get me outa here. I gotta get back 'n take care o' Geneva."

"She don't know those sailors. She don't even know those damn politicians. It's too late fer me to save her innocence, but by God I'll save her from those damn Democrats. The Republicans too. They all got the same idea. They all want my little girl and they can't have her. They c'n have me, 'r Helen, 'r Ruth 'r the others. They c'n have the high yellers if they want 'em, but they can't have Geneva. Get me outa here, I said. Get me outa here."

The Supervisor came in and ordered a jacket. Three days later the Madam roused and said, "What the hell am I doing here? I gotta go home. I gotta go home, I tell you."

She won't though, not very soon. Personally, I think when she does go home she won't be sent, she'll be shipped.

CHAPTER 5

IT IS EVENING AGAIN. We are all in our gowns awaiting nightfall. Our clothes are locked away in the linen room. The nurses are taking the rack of brooms and the scrub buckets and locking them in the hall outside the "hydro" door. Anything which could possibly be used for weapons is kept out of sight as much as possible.

Three of the patients are sleeping heavily under drugs. A third one is singing loudly and tunelessly, another is talking to herself—or rather to the imaginary companions her unreliable mind surrounds her with. Or perhaps it is not an unreliable mind but a very reliable one—it can do for her what a sane mind cannot do for its owner. It can fill a world built of delusion with circumstances and people that are more real than reality.

There is a lovely sunset tonight. Huge clouds are banked against the light but they are not heavy enough to shut the color away. It shines through them and reflects against other soft fleeces, piled high in the air. Everything is saturated in the shimmering, translucent glow. It has a tangible quality that might be caught and held in the fingers. It settles around everything and floats through our windows, transforming everything it touches. Oh, to be able to stand out-of-doors and be bathed in this light from the sunset.

This bright glowing pinkness might be caught and held and

felt in the fingers. A tree at the end of the building makes a beautiful pattern of motion. Its leaves stir and quiver as they feel the light from the sunset slide through them. They turn their smooth side toward it and reflect it a moment. Then dip with the weight of the color so it slides off onto others.

A ray from the sunset has fallen across the face of one of the sleepers, causing it to lose for a moment the heavy, unnatural look the drug left upon it. Instead of being drawn and blue, the ray from the sunset makes it look fresh and pink. The flesh of her cheek looks firm and round and filled with the fresh blood of natural sleeping.

But she moved. The ray no longer leaves its transforming radiance, her head has rolled backwards and is hanging heavily from her neck. Her mouth has fallen open, her tongue lolls thickly, her skin is mottled, clammy and drawn tightly over her features like cold gray rubber. The tip of her nose is very blue; so is her chin and cheek bones where the gray skin is stretched tightest. Her eye-balls are two bulging mounds behind drawn lids—and even the heavy unnatural sleep does not shut away, the memory of the horrors she will again see upon awakening.

The nurses are putting the Student to bed. She goes laggingly, her fresh young body naked; she must be changed through the night as babies are. Her parents come to see her often. They reproach themselves and are torn between despair, hope, fear and waiting. They did not know—how could they know this would happen? But three younger children are not encouraged to be brilliant students.

And now the morning. There was a flood of rain through the night, and the whole world as far as it can be seen from these windows is stirring itself with the business of Spring. Fat robins are tugging at worms, and myriads of other birds flit in and out of the long row of maples stretching down from our windows; but there is rarely enough lull in the noise of this raving for a bird-song to be heard. A mother mallard with a progeny of eight fat ducklings is puddling about in the rainpools and wet grasses. Their freedom makes our confinement unbelievably complete.

The Farm-woman and I have been standing together at a window, looking out at all the beauty flung abroad by Spring. I felt her hand grip my shoulder and from the pressure of her tense fingers the force of the woman herself flowed into me.

"Look outside, there," she commanded me in a low, tense voice, "and see what you see. How pretty it all is! Spring is here and everything is starting to grow. Look inside here and see what happens to people who are shut away from everything they want. God made days like this for people to work and plant things, and tend them and watch them grow. I want to tell you something," she turned toward me and I met her eyes squarely, they were steady, calm and unflinching—and they opened a vista for me to see far into her life.

"Listen; I have stood being shut up just as long as I can. I cannot go on any longer. I know there have been times when it has had to be but they have kept me shut up here months at a time, when I could have been free. But they would not let me go. 'In a little while you will be better; in a little while you will be all right, in a little while you can go home.' I can't stand this concrete floor any longer. They told me last Spring I could go home. And every hour I was ready. The whole year has passed—and now it is Spring again and they do not intend to release me."

"All these years they have just been putting me off; anything they want to tell us is all right; for we do not matter. They were just stringing me along. At last, when I knew it; you know what happened. I had to be tied down again. You know how that is. Now, I know I can never go back to my home."

"I dream of my garden every night—and little chickens hatching. Last night, I dreamed of an old Dominick hen I killed sixteen years ago, because I could not keep her out of my garden. They did not let me go in time to make a garden this year, I cannot stand it any longer. They will never let me go now—for I cannot live through the long years of waiting they insist on. The garden I made the spring I killed the old hen is the last garden I shall ever make—and I hope I won't be alive to worry about it next year."

I floundered for something to say—but there was nothing I could say to bring any comfort. The quietness and conviction of her speech silenced any remonstrance before it was spoken. There was dignity about her, making any opinion I might have seem gauche and callow. She was looking through these bars and longing for the swing of her hoe when I was yet playing kid games in school. I find myself wishing with her that if the need she feels for freedom cannot be granted—and I know she is right in thinking it will not be—that Death will come for her quickly.

She is such a strange person, so poised, serene and soft spoken today as she moves in the "hydro." It is hard to connect her with the same person who lay for weeks in a strait-jacket, raving her lungs out in the pain of her madness. It is hard to believe the soft voice in which she spoke to me this morning has another vocabulary filled with shrieking profanities and strident obscenities.

Today as she moves about there is a dignity and poise and control within her which was completely lost a few weeks ago.

I still am not sure she is the same person. Today she stands erect and moves with a steady step. Her gorgeous auburn hair is held in a great burnished coil at the back of her neck. Her dress is neat and clean (she made it herself, down here, because she did not like the ill-fitting, nondescript garments). It fits her and hangs evenly almost to her ankles, and is molded to the ample spread of her hips, shoulders and bosom.

Just now she is going about her work at the serving table, beating up an egg-nog for the Skeleton, who is standing across the table from her, with her gown ripped from hem to neck as usual. She has braced her hands against the edge of the table and is stretching the bony length of her body across it so her face is very close to the others.

The Skeleton is shrieking and howling that she cannot drink the egg-nog—and is pleading between shrieks for the other not to fix it for her. But the beating and mixing and stirring continues as she watches each movement, her shrieks becoming wilder and wilder. First she started out pleading for it not to be mixed at all, then that there not be a whole egg put into it, then not a whole cup of milk nor a whole spoonful of sugar. And since the other ignored her altogether, and went serenely on with the mixing, her shrieks grew louder and louder and now they are literally tearing her throat out and deafening the rest of us. But the Farm-woman has finished the mixing and is holding the cup out towards her. She will not take it. Her hands are gripping each other and the whiteness of the straining knuckles make them look more like bones than ever. She is stark, stark mad with despair and gives voice to the most fantastic assertions.

"I can't take it, I can't take it, can't you see I can't take it. My throat has been cut—see; so I cannot swallow! My throat has been cut, my tongue is cut out, my lips are cut off!! I cannot swallow, I can't even speak—(she makes guttural noises to prove it). See, oh please, please, *please*—can't you see I can't do it? My tongue is gone—see?" (She opened her mouth wide to show us).

Now she is waving her arms wildly and howling. But the egg-nog is ready and the other is reaching into the cabinet to get the peg. Bones is shrieking louder and louder. They stand there together, one poised and serene; while the other shrieks louder and louder.

"Take it—take it—take it or I'll call the nurse."

There is no escaping it. The distress of the other has mounted until her eyes are all run together and do not look like human eyes. The nurse has come to the table and taken the cup and peg from the other and has offered Bones the choice of drinking the egg and milk or of having it poured down her. Her eyes oscillate wildly from the peg to the cup and back to the peg. She reaches a claw-like hand for the lesser of the two evils, but cannot bring herself to the point of taking it into her hand, much less drinking the contents. She draws back as though the cup contained deadly poison. She feels nothing but terror.

It is so senseless—but it is very real to her, so real that it has run her eyes together and given her features the gray pallor of dying. The nurse makes a threatening gesture, Bones takes the cup craftily and tries to dash into the stool-room. But they head her off. She is trapped with the deadly thing in her hand—and no chance to dispose of it unless she drinks it down.

The nurse is saying, "Drink it or I'll use the peg." Bones' claw-like hands grip the cup. She holds it away from her and the shrieks that come from her straining throat lift her body on tip-toe. The peg has come closer so she lifts the cup to her lips—but there are no words in the world to describe the look on her face. She took one mighty gulp—and strangles on the shrieks which started out as she did it.

"O-o-o-o-o-o-o-lp!!! O, I can't do it! Please, Please can't you see I can't do it?"

But the peg is there, ready, so she tries once again but fear is clutching her throat so it really will not respond to the motion of swallowing. It can only obey her impulse to scream and the noise comes up and mingles in the milk that fills her mouth. But because her throat is wide open to make an exit for her screams, the milk trickles coolly around her livid terror and finds its way to her stomach. Now it is finished—and she is panting and shrieking. Now she is charging madly about. The last meal was the same as this one—and the next will be a repetition with scant variations.

She stopped her charging and stands beside me, still shrieking. She is shaking my chair and jerking it about, so when this sentence is finished no one will be able to read it, but it does not matter.

I am helpless to help her and stark mad myself or I would not feel as I do toward her. The nurse is standing over us; she who shrieks madness; and I who write it in order not to. The nurse is telling her to be quiet if she does not want a jacket. But she has no comprehension of anything said to her and has singled me out; I cannot refuse her, though I know I can't help her.

"I want to tell you, please let me tell you. They made me drink milk, and I can't even swallow. Please won't you tell them I cannot swallow—won't you please tell them?"

"They do not believe me when I tell them my throat has been cut and my lips are cut off and my tongue is cut out. I tried to tell them—but they wouldn't listen. Please; won't you tell them? See, my tongue is gone, and I cannot speak. I can't speak a word."

I tried once again to help her, "All right. I'll try to help if you will keep still and listen a minute." But she tried all the harder to convince me of the fantastic things she believed about herself.

When she saw she had my attention, she clamped her hands tightly before her; but before she was finished, she was gripping my shoulders so I could not escape, as fantastic ideas poured from her in a flood. She wound up the endless account of her horrors with the assertion "I can't eat—I can't sleep—I can't sit—I can't spit—I have no tongue!"

When I asked if that was the only thing the matter with her she said it was not nearly all. Then started again at the beginning. By the time she had finished the second account she was quieter and I had the vain hope, as she calmed down a little, that maybe another idea could be wedged cross-wise into all the confusion and horror.

I listened while she finished her ritual—and by that time her horrified eyes had lost some of the look they had when she started and I tried to get to her.

She followed me—and I gave all I had of reason and insight and kindness, but it was not enough to benefit her. I thought I was making some progress but made the fatal error of running smack into one of her phobias. I lifted her hand and laid her bone-like fingers against her strained neck-tendon. (Perhaps it was the knife-like edge of it that gave her the idea.)

When I asked her to tell me what she felt there under her fingers she answered with a shriek of stark terror as her eyes dilated wildly.

"Yes—yes—it is so. I can feel it. Oh, I can feel it! See, here it is, here. My throat's been cut—my throat is cut—My Throat is Cut!"

I had failed.

It was the Farm-woman who initiated me to the shocks that I must adjust myself to, if I were going to live in the "hydro." She started my education early in the first few hours I was here.

I was all eyes and expectancy anyway, and felt nothing but the shrinking revulsion most people feel toward the violently demented, as at that time I was not quite one of them. Since then I have learned to know them better; you live very close to your fellows in an insane asylum.

When I was sent down here, I was being given medicine, for a shrieking pain in my shoulder which the Doctors thought was hysteria. Because it is harder to reach a warped mind with potions and powders, and because they really wanted to help me, they prescribed a sodium salicilate compound. Of course, they did not tell me what it was, merely sent the bottle to the nurse.

She called me to her, measured the dose to be given me and said, "Swallow it." I recognized the flavor, I had taken it before for the same trouble.

The first evening I was in the "hydro" the nurse called out to me to bring a spoon and come to the linen room.

I went to the serving table and asked the Farm-woman for it. She was instantly on guard as though I had asked for enough nitroglycerine to blow her up.

"What do you want with a spoon?"

"The nurse told me to get it and come in there to her."

"Now you know she did not tell you to get a spoon. You are just lying; you'd better get away from here!"

I did not quite know what to do in a case like that—for the Farm-woman had charge of the serving table. She was glaring at me in a manner that made me very undecided. But with her narrowed eyes on me she asked, "What does the nurse want you to bring a spoon for?"

"Why, to measure my medicine with."

"How come you're taking medicine?"—suspiciously.

"The Doctor prescribed it."

"What is it?"—narrowly.

"Why—I don't know exactly what all it is—but mostly sodi—."

"You lie! You lie! The soda's up here in the shelves and I take care of them. You're just a low down liar! You can't have any soda and you can't have any spoon and if you don't get away from here, I'll throw this hot water on you and scald the sneaky, lying hide off you."

By that time I knew I did not want any spoon or any soda or anything else. I backed out of reach of the scalding water. She had it aimed toward me and was just waiting one more remark to let me have it.

The nurse called to her to shut up and give me a spoon. I sidled back to get it as courageously as I could while she cursed me in a vicious undertone and kept her hand threateningly near her weapon—the hot water.

Next morning she was mopping the dormitory. Claw-belly was tied; as she usually is; but was in a very happy mood and singing. The Farm-woman told her to hush but she paid no attention. The other spoke to her more commandingly. Still she gave no sign of hearing, and kept right on with her singing.

The Farm-woman spoke a third time in such a manner that even anyone as demented as Claw-belly could not fail to catch the import. She was being told to shut up in no uncertain man-

/78/

ner but raised her head from her pillow and swore good naturedly at the Farm-woman.

That made the Farm-woman thoroughly angry and she came striding down the aisle like an avenging Fury. Her lips were drawn in a snarl. There was a flush in her cheeks and a glint in her eyes that boded no good to the other. When she reached Claw-belly's bed she stood and glared down upon her, giving vent to a scalding stream of profanity more inclusive and expressive than anything I had ever heard in my life, up to that time at least.

"I told you to hush!—And you're Going to hush! You sniveling daughter of a hell bound whore!"

Where-upon she seized the business end of the sopping mop she had been using and stuffed as much of it into the other's mouth as it would hold, and washed her face, none too gently with the rest of it; accompanying the whole operation with curses.

When the nurses came and took the Farm-woman away, Claw-belly, whose mouth had been stopped and whose face had been washed, gave vent to a stream of profanity classic in its purity. That is, it was pure in the sense that it was unmixed with anything else—and it was so heart felt and expressive it made the other woman's raging expressions seem dumb and speechless by comparison. It was in a class by itself, nowhere in the world could there be other speech like it. It was an exclamation point at the end of the ultimate!

The mouth-gagging, face washing episode marked the end of the Farm-woman's self control. She who had waited and held herself steady as the weeks wore into months and the months had rolled themselves into years, cracked. She was tied down before that day was finished.

She lay for weeks in a strait-jacket, as her frustration rolled out into the world in a stream of raving. None of the words she knew were strong enough to carry it. It became shrieks and howls that were the starkest madness imaginable.

I was given her job at the serving table. She hated me passionately because of it. Her curses were violent things to hear, every time she caught sight of me. She had one pet epithet viler than the others and reserved it for me. I had taken the job which; as long as she was able to hold; meant she could hope to go free when her people came for her.

Because she had lost it she lost all control of herself also—she knew she could never go free and her madness became such a driving force within her she could do nor say nothing terrible enough to justify it, nor satisfy it or fulfill the claim it had upon her.

She was kept locked in the side-room most of the time. One night she managed to wriggle out of her jacket, climbed up on her bed and tore the light fixture from the ceiling. I was awakened to help put her back into her jacket. It was an eerie sensation to feel the tenseness and uncertainty the nurses felt about unlocking the door.

They stood several minutes debating whether the three of us could handle her. She was stark mad, free, and would fight like a tiger. The room was in darkness so she could not be seen through the small, grated peep-hole, they could only suspect she was crouched in a corner waiting to spring upon the first one who came through the door, with the heavy porcelain fixture as a weapon—and that she would fight to kill.

They decided we should all rush her. They flung the door open and caught her before she had a chance to strike. But we could not hold her. There was a queer elusiveness about her smooth, flexed muscles, and though her flesh felt firm when we touched it, we could not grasp her in a grip she did not shake off. We found whenever our hands seemed to be closing firmly upon her, she'd manage to slip away from us and our hands would be gripping the empty air. She seemed to be everywhere, and nowhere. We struggled in silence but as first one and then another held her for one straining second, her breathing began to be heavy.

There was something so tense and eerie about fighting there in the half-dark with a maniac who made no out-cry and whose smooth firm flesh seemed to evaporate when we caught it, that I do not wonder now, why superstitious people believe firmly that Madness is something connected with Satan. But if we could not hold her, neither did we allow her freedom to have a clear swing at striking.

She put all she had into the struggle and soon wore herself down to a strength we could handle. Her breath was coming in great sobbing gasps when we finally got her into the jacket. Our breathing also was labored, but not as hers was. She had fought with grim desperation for a chance to give action to the terrible forces of Madness. The raging urge within her knew no law except the blind necessity of the violence it was set upon doing.

Madness will sacrifice its victim gladly in torment if it can find some means of expression. It knows nothing of fear or disaster—would even enter death gladly in the hope of finding an outlet for itself in the dying. It is stronger than the will to live—or the law of self preservation. It is the law of self preservation, run amuck among forces it knows nothing about.

A few nights later the nurses woke me to help with her. Again she had wriggled out of her jacket, but this time she did not fight so desperately. When we went in we found she had ripped her pillow open and strewn the feathers all over the room.

She was standing by her bed, curling her toes and rubbing her feet in them, ecstatically. But when we began to clean up the mess of feathers—we found we must clean up a worse mess beneath them. Dust-pans have strange uses in an insane asylum.

In those days I wonder why the nurses felt so sad at seeing her so. Always they spoke of her as being such a "sweet" person—and I had seen nothing about her that could be called "sweet" as I understood the word. So I wondered and asked them.

One of them told me, "Oh, she is not like this when she is herself. She is really one of the nicest patients we've ever had but she is a devil when she gets 'disturbed.'"

The days that followed her crash were the days which preceded my own. We became very good friends in the interim and sought each other's companionship. The choice was partly from necessity, for at that time we were the only two patients in the Hydro not in the throes of their Madness.

In the intermission we have sat together and talked long and wonderingly of many things. The eternal Why? Why? of such things. She has opened vistas for me to see far into her life—and when you know a person as well as I learned to know her—the knowledge brings with it an affection real and gripping.

I found we have enough in common to be friends in the truest sense of the word. When friendship comes all curiosity gives place to understanding. Their very failures and weaknesses endear them to you.

One day I asked her why she had torn the light fixture out of the ceiling and if she remembered doing it.

"Sure I do—and I did it because I wanted to do something

mean and that was all I could think of. I'm glad now I did not hurt any of you when you came to tie me down again. Though at the time there was nothing I wanted to do quite so much as to kill all of you!"

"But," I asked, "how about the feathers?"

"I wanted something to stand on. I wanted earth! Ground! But I could not have it and that was all I could get, so I took it. I know it made them all mad but I could not help it. I had to have something."

Then I asked her why we felt so toward things—and her answer was so to the point it left me staggered with the truth of her statement.

"I don't know—I guess we're just plain crazy."

CHAPTER 6

"NOW, GET IN there and shut up," said a nurse as she shoved an attractive young woman through the door to the "Hydro." I looked up from "Shakespeare" and saw a woman of about thirty-five being forced toward a bed.

As the nurse pushed her along she protested violently, "Quit shoving, damn you. I'm going but I hate to be pushed, cut it out before I yank you bald headed and make you wish you'd stayed on the farm."

The nurse only laughed and said, "You're not much crazier than I am. Go along now and get ready for a bath." As soon as the nurse stopped pushing, the woman sat down on a bed and started removing her clothes.

"That's a good-looking carcass you've got there," said the nurse as she took the clothing preparatory to locking it up.

"Yeah," answered the woman, "that's my legacy."

"Legacy?" queried the nurse. "I see the 'legs' part all right but how come you say that?"

"Oh, that's a long story. Too damn long, if you ask me, and besides you're too young to know. Wait till you grow up and maybe some of the big girls'll tell you about the stork which carries the same kind of kids to the same kind of families generation after generation and then you'll know."

"I s'pose you're a direct descendant of the Queen of Sheba.

I hear she was quite a gal in her day, or maybe I shoulda said, in her nights."

"Queen of Sheba, that amateur, hell, my ancestors, or my ancestresses at least, probably had to teach her where to put her perfume. Queen of Sheba, why old Cleo or Catherine or Borgia were all mere infants at the 'Art' compared to the people I come from," exclaimed the woman whom I later learned to think of and call the Schizo.

"Okay, okay, let's get this bath over. We got Napoleons 'n Josephines, and Shakespeares, might as well have Cleopatra's consultor," answered the nurse. "I don't think we need any mummies, but we could use a change from the zombies in here."

"Never you mind," said Schizo, "the only thing this body is wrapped up in is its Art, and you can spell that with long hair and a Capital 'A'."

They moved off toward the bathtub and I continued with old Willie, The Bard.

When you are crazy you see things—sometimes delicious things—which poor dumb sanity misses completely. Because sanity is slow, stupid and reasonable. It does not have the swift, sudden flashes of seeing which are one of the compensations of Madness. When you know you are crazy you do not have to appear logical to anyone, least of all, to yourself. So, because I am Shakespeare and because he has the memory of a former existence in which he was a genius; he does not blush at finding beauty where others miss it.

Today is scrub day—and Shakespeare and I have been helping with it. Shakespeare—grubbed up in a scrub-bucket!—I have scrubbed miles of floors in my life, but not until I became insane enough to claim Shakespeare, was I ever able to find sparkling beauty in scrubbing—that most plebian of all grubby chores. But Shakespeare taught me some new tricks about it. He found an entire symphony orchestra in such material as soapsuds and sun-light and cement.

Comparing nuts to soap bubbles—yes, we are very insane, Shakespeare. But there was also much beauty in the dance of one of the patients—such beauty as those who study art all their lives are not able to catch and interpret.

Tell how she stood at her bedside with her hair all tumbled from sleeping—amusing herself by stroking the little grey kitten she played with. How the kitten stretched a paw through the foot rail and plucked at a flower in the print of her pajamas. How she lifted her eyes to the morning, her throat athrob with the life tingling and thrilling within her. How she flung her arms upward in a tense gesture of greeting; without conscious volition on her part; it was the soul buried beneath her warped thinking which flung her arms upward to greet the bright sunlight.

The sun etched her smooth amber body in an outline of fire. It spun her short tousled hair into a magnificent headdress of gold and gave her bright print pajamas colors more barbarously pagan than any modern dyestuffs could leave in them.

She was the living image of an ancient sun-goddess and fulfilled the rest of the ritual. Her steps at first were uncertain but as her feet found the rhythm her whole glowing body responded as it moved to the tempo of a wild pagan harmony which only her soul was hearing.

Her feet moved to it, her arms were extended—suspended in it. It carried her backward into the dim past and things of forgotten ages. She had the spirit of a pagan sun-goddess and was dancing a dance the world has forgotten for ages. No conscious study of expression could have expressed the meaning and movement that her flowing members depicted—in madness.

It was a fierce need for expression which moved her and as she felt the rhythm of the madness she moved so her steps became faster and faster, but always she danced in the sunlight and wore the exotic costume of a pagan. The soft fluffy kitten, her partner—filled in the contrast in pattern; for always it held her interest.

The nurses came running and told her to stop it—but she could not hear them because she was held in the grip of her madness and could do nothing but follow. They caught and tried to hold her, but could not stop her.

The dance was upon her, she could no more have stopped it than she could her heart in its beating.

Nothing can stop such fierce need for expression but the brute force of superior numbers, for the need she felt is madness. They brought a strait-jacket but by that time she had delivered her soul of the burden and stood panting before them —so they did not tie her.

Truly such beautiful dancing is seldom seen in a lifetime, even though it was staged in a bug-house before breakfast; with an unappreciative audience composed only of nuts and nurses who threatened a strait-jacket.

They can say what they please but I know the dance helped her. She has been quiet since, not with the silence that results from the suppression which is our portion here—but with the quietness that results from satisfactory expression. For the dance she did was more beautiful than she knew. Though she did not do it to meet the approval of anyone, or give anyone pleasure, or a chance to applaud her for creating something of beauty.

The nurses who threatened to tie her did not know there are

people in the world who pay fancy prices to see exhibitions of dancing which do not approach the magnificent beauty she depicted. They would call her an artist and lay down a tribute of all the world has to offer in applause and appreciation. As it is, she is only a nut in a bug-house--from whose mouth a tooth has been broken because she is so violently insane she must be fed by "pegging." And that is that, Shakespeare; you are a nut yourself for thinking such heretical thoughts.

One of the patients from upstairs just now passed the window and waved to me gaily, swinging on in a great elation that she had been chosen for the menial task of trash carrying. It means a chance to breathe deeply, a few breaths of air not filtered through the bars of confinement.

It means she has angled long and patiently for the office, and has waged a campaign greater than seems worthy of the small reward going with it.

She is the "original patent" nut—and I wish she would do something or other to get transferred to the "hydro," if she could do it without going off the deep end. I would hate to see that happen to her, but I like her very much and would enjoy her companionship.

She has had much experience in these institutions and has told me much of her life.

There are deep white scars circling each of her wrists—scars that were made by steel manacles which held her for two years in an asylum in another State.

She is an accomplished pianist—though the things she plays are so highly classical few of her audience appreciate her accomplishment. In fact, her playing sounds so loud to others who are trying to sleep, the night supervisor laid down some rules about when she could play. The nervous surge of energy through her fingers prevents her from playing in anything but the loudest fortissimo.

She is such a vivid, stimulating personality—and has such a humorous slant on things that life can never be monotonous around her. In fact, she is so like a pet monkey there is no telling one minute, what she will devise to disrupt the peace of the next.

Her husband is also an inmate in another institution in another State—and I have a breath-taking wonder as I think of the possibility for living that those two have passed on to a daughter now kept by a relative. The mother is in one institution—"hyper-kinetic"—and the father a dipsomaniac in another.

The Medicine-maker called me to her bed just now, to share something so exciting she could not refrain from sharing it. She could not place a finger on her lips to warn me to silence—but a tense shake of the head and a sibilant "Ssh" were convincing enough she wanted me to be secret.

I went to her bedside, wondering, as her eyes were glittering with excitement. When I was within easy ear-shot of her whispering voice, she said from one corner of her mouth:

"Sh-sh-sh! Don't say anything about it to the nurses—but a patient is running away! See! There she goes—Ssh! Let her get started—don't say a word about it. Go back over there and act like you don't know anything. Maybe she can make it. Oh, I hope she does! Won't they be mad when they find out about it? Don't you dare say a word. Won't they be mad. Oh, won't they be mad!"

I looked outside but saw no one who looked like a patient. She seems excited enough to be having a delusion—she is quivering with it—; her eyes are still sparkling like fire-works—and her cheeks are flushed crimson. Her body is stretched tense and rigid; her pulses are pounding madly—I can see them race through her throat. Her mouth is a livid gash, white at the edges. Never have I seen anyone so excited—yet making no out-cry!

She must be reliving a memory of her own mad dash for freedom. That happened before I came here—but the patients up on the ward told me the story. She worked out all the details carefully, and on arising one morning, complained of being cold and asked permission to wear a coat from the locker. She had wormed herself into the good graces of the nurse on the ward and was chosen for the morning chore of trash carrying.

When she got to the burner, instead of turning back to the door where the nurse waited, she dashed off around the corner of the building, and the patient who was with her dashed in hot pursuit after her.

Those upstairs who were watching saw the fluttering dress of the other patient; a great cry went up that she was the one making the break for freedom.

By the time the Medicine-maker had reached the road she had far outdistanced the other, but a car was drawing to a stop in her path. The two men in it had taken the situation in at a glance and climbed out to meet her.

She saw their intention and, without slacking pace, swooped up two rocks from the roadside. With her crude weapons she tried to dispose of the men who attempted to gum up her plans. But they caught her and brought her back to the office, where one of them was given treatment for cuts and bruises. She had smashed his face in.

I suppose the State paid his garage bill. She'd hurled one of the rocks through his windshield. I don't know who paid his hospital bills, after all, he wasn't crazy. Or was he?

Though that escape happened months ago, she has not often been out of a strait-jacket since. The attendants do not interfere with her. They leave her to her silence, and do not often speak to her.

Her hatred has grown and expanded until it fills everything she has ever had knowledge of. And truly all the horrors of the world have not been experienced by anyone who has not seen the Medicine-maker's eyes. It is impossible to look into them and not feel the flesh shrink in revulsion from something that cannot be analyzed—only felt—and fled from.

The place is in more of an uproar than usual tonight. Everyone gets more nervous as night advances—and by suppertime those who are raving have whooped up the racket until everybody is either raving, or wanting to.

The Farm-woman is again lying on her bed with her head covered. She and the Student and the Musician and Shakespeare and I are the only ones quiet—and Shakespeare and I are raving on paper—so I do not know that we are to be excepted.

The Musician is a girl who has spent most of her life studying music—and was well on the way to recognition. Now it is finished, I suppose, forever. She sits for hours and hours, as does the Student. Neither of them ever move or give any indication they have consciousness of life. However, the Musician, if stirred from her inertia by another will complete whatever she was set to doing with frenzied motion, and as soon as it is finished settle back into the first inertia, not to move again until someone starts her at something else.

She is such a strange person. Just now one of the night nurses started her back to her bed. She rushed toward it in breathless haste, her arms swinging loosely. But the hopeless inertia that holds her in its paralyzing grasp cannot be broken.

The days roll into weeks, into months, into years. An ever widening gulf between her and her piano, as the sound of music now drives her mad. The despair she feels is graven deeply in furrows between her wild eyes; and she is not yet out of her twenties.

A little patient who was at one time in the "hydro" but was transferred back to the ward where I had been told me a story about the Musician which amused her greatly. This little patient was tied down in a jacket like most of the others. Bones and the Musician were not. Bones, with all her howling and raving, is perfectly harmless and is only tied down when they must restrain her to give her worn-out body some rest. So these two were loose in the "hydro."

The night nurses had drawn the serving table into the dormitory to use as a desk. This night they had brought two candy bars with them and placed them on the table while they went about the work of attending the patients. When they finished and were seating themselves at the table they noticed one of the candy bars was missing. A hunt failed to locate it, so they accused Bones of taking it.

The patient said Bones did not take it. She had seen the Musician dash up and snatch it. But the nurses did not believe her and thought Bones was guilty. Bones thought they were planning some fresh torture and she shrieked and pleaded before them. The little patient feared the nurses down here madly but came to the defense of the innocent and gave voice to loud protest which went unheard in the general confusion. Midway of the uproar, when the nurses were concerned with Bones only, the guilty one dashed up and grabbed the other candy-bar.

The little patient who told it let out such a shout they turned in time to see the culprit dash back to bed. They sprang after her in hot pursuit, catching her midway of the aisle, but when they searched her they found no trace of the candy, not even the cellophane wrapper! For that matter, though they searched her bed carefully, they found no trace of the first wrapper, either —so they came to the conclusion that she who never moved unless started in motion, had been prodded into action by her craving for candy. The patient who told me about it was convulsed with laughter and wound up by lamenting the fact the candy was eaten with the flavor wrapped in water-proof cellophane.

The Puckish face of Humor is often seen in the "hydro" grinning impishly from behind some fold in the sable draperies of madness, who sits here among us, somber and brooding, eyeing us grimly—and waiting.

Bones is the one who most often provokes mirth among us. When a patient was transferred to the hospital, almost dead from raving—her bed was filled by another before the nurse had returned from the errand. The new patient was in a strait-jacket. For hours her protests filled the "hydro." Hour after hour after hour, a monotonous repetition of phrases that did not change in inflection or meaning, until at last it resembled nothing but the high-pitched squeak of machinery, badly in need of oiling.

"Release me—release me—in the name of Jesus, release me—Rele-e-ease me—re-le-e-ease me, in-the-name-of Jesus, rele-e-ease me." Hour after hour until our ears ached with monotony.

The Mother, on the bed adjoining her, was not tied at the time. She hates a strait-jacket so much herself she can hardly endure to see another in one. (In fact, that is why she herself is kept tied so much of the time.)

When she is loose, she goes around untying others. She had resisted the monotonous appeal for several hours—but could endure it no longer. She leaned from her bed and started untying the piece of machinery which needed oiling. Even while she was at it, the other didn't stop squeaking, "Release me, release me—in the name of Jesus—release me."

The nurse saw the Mother and brought a strait-jacket for her. They tied the first one back. While they were at it, the voice did not lose a squeak. When they were finished, they turned and tied the Mother down, too. She voiced her protests with a racket like a boiler exploding.

When the nurses were finished with tying the Mother, and her fury had settled enough to allow her to speak words, she said, with her red hair standing on end and her cheeks puffing with the panting breath of her anger:

"Shut up—Shut up—*Shut—up*—I want you to *shut up!* I tried to 'release you, in the name of Jesus'—and look what happened to me!"

That tickled Bones. She was lying on a bed next to the Mother. She started laughing. The Mother divided her wrath between the two of them, but nothing checked Bones and her laughter. She laughed and she laughed. She rolled over in bed and laughed. She drew her knobby knees up to the tip of her sharp chin and laughed. She got up on her knees and hid her face down between them and laughed. Every sharp bone and angle in her whole body thrust a barb through the mirth and became anchored in it. The chattering joints which held her rattling bones together were almost uncoupled with it, but still she laughed. She shifted from one grotesque position to another, and finally, just in time to keep from falling apart altogether, she rolled over on her back, her ripped gown revealed her quaking abdomen, convulsed with more animation than any other part of her clattering anatomy. She clawed the air helplessly—and laughed, and her laughter was so contagious it swept among us like a virulent epidemic. We all laughed at the way she was laughing and forgot all the humor which had produced it.

Nothing I have ever seen or heard is as funny as the "Skeleton" when she is laughing. No one had ever before seen her so much as smile. The nurses stood watching—and were infected with the contagion.

When it was finished, she rose from her bed, wiped the tears from her eyes with the backs of her talon-like hands and ambled off into the stool-room. She came back in a moment, still chuckling, with the bed-pan carried loosely before her. She ambled up to the piece of machinery which had not lost a creak in its squawking. Pulling the sheet from around it, she solemnly slipped the bed-pan beneath it, saying, "Here Sister—use this 'in the name of Jesus.'"

That was the cue for the way to manage the other. She would do nothing that was not prefaced with the "Name of Jesus" ritual. Whether it was water or food or drugs or a bath, she would have nothing that was not offered by saying "Take this—in the name of Jesus." Bones enjoyed feeding her and would preface each bite she offered with the phrase.

Bones' laugh had helped her greatly. She went about for days after, in so much better spirits it seemed likely that she would be transferred from the hydro. But at last she lost all the benefit from it and was seen to slip slowly into her old despair. But she did not forget how; like magic, the formula of the "Name of Jesus" had worked on the woman.

Several weeks later, when one of the nurses was trying to get another patient to do something or other, Bones stopped long enough in her endless pacing and raving to cock her head to one side and listen. When she had taken in the situation, she stalked up to the nurse, with her face thrust forward and offered her solemn contribution of helpfulness—"Did you try 'In the name of Jesus' on her?"—and turned another laugh loose in the hydro that she did not share in.

The "Schizo" has been here for weeks now and I don't see why she is kept in the hydro. For that matter, I don't see why she is kept in the asylum at all, but then, I'm crazy, too, remember?

She goes about assisting the nurses with feeding, changing beds, and generally making herself useful.

Her only signs of insanity are occasional spells of brooding. At these times she is very cantankerous. If disturbed, she is apt to lash out harshly at anyone who speaks to her or interrupts her train of thought.

I spoke to her one day as she lay in a jacket the Doctor had ordered because she had slapped the Pagan when this beautiful automaton crept close to her and attempted to stroke her golden hair.

No one knows why anything which even remotely resembles the sunlight affects the Pagan so. It just does; and that's that.

As she lay there, not struggling as we usually do, against the jacket, I asked her, "Why are you here? You're not insane. Did some lawyer get you out of a murder or something with one of those 'temporary insanity' pleas?" And she told me just what she had told the nurse the day she came.

"It's my legacy, my inheritance. Now get the hell away before I bust out of this cocoon and crown you!" So—I went back to sly old Shakespeare.

The little brown "Field-mouse" just now stopped behind and picked up one of the sheets I have written. It is not the first time she has done it—it is a ritual she goes through almost every time she passes. She is such an odd little creature—and so pathetic. To see the pain she suffers when her mind comes to grips with reality—is to feel grateful to Madness for giving her even the fantastic escape through delusion.

To see her lie grieving for days at a time because she is forsaken by friends and family alike and because even her children have sent no word to her for over six years, is to feel glad she can escape the unendurable pain of it all by slipping out into delusion.

We are abnormal people—crazy—insane. We are depressed or morbid or violent or vicious—those are the usual adjectives. But because we are still human beings (opinions of doctors and nurses to the contrary) there is a little which is horrible, some tragic, more which is pathetic, some ridiculous—and much that is very lovely.

Just now the Field-mouse perused the sheet held before her—(up-side-down—but it did not matter, her eyesight is too poor to read, even with glasses. Besides her education did not include learning even the rudiments of reading or writing). But those handicaps are surmounted, brushed aside, dismissed as wholly irrelevant, by a mind which must hurdle through madness, every obstacle in its way. She held the sheet raptly before her, her eyes glowing very brightly, as she said to me:

"Ah! I am so glad to know you are a writer for I too, do things that are different. I am the greatest opera star in the world! I have sung before kings—and all the great of the earth. I rode up before them on a snow-white horse—and sang to them such songs as had never been heard, they called me the greatest singer in the world. See this star in my forehead? It was there when I was born, a sign. A sign that I would one day be a great opera star. I sang before them, my songs made me great and famous. When they heard me sing they put gold and diamonds in this star in my forehead and called me the greatest singer the world has ever known."

She went on back to her bed—her flannelette night-gown, dingy, worn and grey from many trips to the laundry, wrapped about her cross-wise, held by a bulging knot tied between one sleeve and the hem at the corner. A fantastic costume, completed by her brown hair hanging, uncombed and matted in a drab mantle almost to her waist. Now she is singing in a tuneless monologue as she looks through a window. I caught a few words of the song, something about, "Washing her cats and dogs in Ivory soap, till they are all very white and clean—then taking them into the woods to hang them in willow trees till they dry."

The nurses hate her singing, they scold her incessantly about it. They have learned she sings more when she can see out a window, so they keep all the windows in her line of vision down and will not let her stand at one.

Even with her crazy singing—she makes far less noise than most of the others. It never gets higher in pitch than a tuneless monologue, almost under her breath. But one day they were more impatient with her than usual and had closed all the windows with a bang. Yet with all their scolding they could not make her hush, so they threatened her with a "sick" hypo.

She faced them as her rebellion burst into flame within her.

She had an expression like a trapped animal facing its captors. It was madness which gave her the courage to face them—a courage that transformed her trapped helplessness into something like triumph. And Madness gave her powers of expression that were magnificent.

"Bring on your sick hypos—twenty grains each, two at a time! Bring on your strait-jackets—make them of iron! Put more bars at the windows; stronger locks on the doors! Lock me in! Shut me up! Send me out of the world altogether! You have taken my home; you have taken my husband; you have taken my children away from me! Are you such fools you still think you have the power to do anything to me that will matter. No—No—All has been done that could be done—and a sick hypo means nothing! Bring them on! Triple strength, three at a time, and a strait-jacket with them! You do not have the courage to kill me; that would be treating me kindly; but you are fools to think a sick hypo will matter!"

They brought her the hypo. I sat by her bed-side and watched her. A green pallor of death spread over her features. The flesh of her cheeks shrank away from nostrils that were pinched and dilated. Great beads of sweat oozed from her skin; coldly; and rolled away slowly, as though they were almost congealed into ice. Her eye-balls bulged in their sockets, pinched into peaks behind the drawn lids, closed like green shutters, but shutters too thin and transparent to hide what went on behind them— they clung to the rocking eye-balls rolling slowly behind them. Presently she began to retch; her nausea so great a sound did not leave her.

I lifted her hair and cleaned the floor around her bed. Presently she slept. When she awoke, I could not bring enough water to quench her burning thirst. She complained of her head and nose itching. As her own hands were tied I did what I could to bring comfort to her—but did not have enough strength in my fingers to relieve the itching. I held the rough edge of the bed-spread tight, so she might rub the twitching tip of her nose against it. They kept her tied down for days, and I tried to render what comfort I could.

When my turn came and I was tied down and given a sick hypo, she repaid me many times over for the consideration shown her. She sat beside me; would not leave me; and was patience itself in trying to minister to me. It was then I learned such shallow treatment as scratching can in no wise relieve the itching left along the nerves from a sick hypo. And water will not quench the thirst brought on by it.

At that time she too, was heavily under the influence of other drugs; but she would get up from her bed every few minutes and go staggering and falling to the water cooler to bring me many cups; full when she started, but by the time she reeled down the length of the aisle back to me, they were almost empty.

So, because we have been through the same things together; have stood by and helped each other, I have enough affection to make me resent the way they treat her. She is not inarticulate about her friendship. She has many odd ways to express it. I never take a bath that she does not slip up and get into the tub behind me. I never hear her; but the first thing I know, she is in there with me, bathing.

Several times every day she will creep up behind me and throw her arms tightly around me—and every day she goes through the ritual of examining what I have written. There is something so pathetic about the way she has responded to my blunt overtures of kindness, that I must say were motivated at first by curiosity—it makes me feel shame for my motives.

I have never seen her do a thing to another that was at all harmful. She is so little that she could not do anything very bad if she tried. It is just another of the many odd things here which are past understanding. As far as I can tell it all boils down thickly to this one thing; the nurses dislike her. But because I took it upon myself to champion her cause, the nurse to whom I talked gave me some enlightenment when she said indignantly:

"I don't care how mean they treat her—I just hate her and she knows it! Do you notice she never speaks to me when I am down here? Well she'd better not, if she knows what's good for her. She knows better than speak to me! I haven't got a bit of use for her and she knows it!"

My eyes were bulging with amazement; I had never heard a nurse speak so heatedly. Then she told me the story.

"The Field-mouse used to be on 'Three-Building' which she cannot discuss without going completely off into raving. She becomes violently suicidal when she grieves for her children. One night I was left on the ward with a few of the patients while the others went for their supper. I missed the 'Field-mouse' from the group I had herded into the dayhall and when I went to hunt for her, found her in the bath-room."

"I caught her arm and told her to get herself out there with the others. She just stood there and looked at me and laughed that crazy laugh of hers. I saw blood on her mouth and asked her what caused it; I shook her—but she would not answer me. Just stood there and laughed! One of the others came in and found the frames of her glasses on the floor. I ran and called the Doctor. We worked with her nearly all night. She was the bloodiest mess I ever saw! The Doctor did not think she would live at all, I was so mad I could have killed her myself! Doing a thing like that when I was on duty. Do you know what she had done?"

"She ground the lens of her glasses under her heel and ate them on a piece of gingerbread!"

"I don't care how mean they treat her! I hope they kill her! I still hate her!"

That happened several years ago. The Field-mouse has been transferred to the hydro and is watched more closely. She does not wear spectacles—but there is no expiation she can make for her misfortune in being unable to dispose of a life which is more torture to her than death.

I have heard her grieve and pray heartbrokenly to be allowed to die. They can do nothing to make her life endurable. They snatched her back from death and forced her to continue it, and they resent the pitiful escape Madness gives her.

This same nurse told me another story—also involving herself. There was a woman on "Three-Building" who had masturbated till the flesh was torn and bleeding. The Doctor told this nurse to give her a lysol douche. The lysol is in huge hospital size bottles and this nurse was going about the business of preparing the douche when one of the other nurses was attracted by the odd way she went at it. She had filled the douche-bag with the undiluted lysol and was preparing to use it—full strength!

"I didn't know anything about using that stuff. Anyway, it would have been good enough for her if I had used it full strength. Anybody that would do a thing like that!"

This woman is by far the most refined of the women who give themselves to our care. She is a school teacher and works here only during vacations. And for her sake, it is a pity there are not twelve months of school. She is dainty; nice; right. To be a nurse of any sort requires a sweep of sympathy too broad to be contained within the narrow confines of "niceness," as she typifies the word. A certain un-niceness is the first requisite of those who care for the insane; both for our comfort and their peace of mind.

This woman has a shuddering revulsion at the boisterous revelations of nakedness, both physical and psychic; seen in the hydro and "Three-Building." She told me she had a shrinking dread each morning when she went to the office for orders and always heaved a great sigh of relief when her work was to be on one of the better wards.

CHAPTER 7

THE MEDICINE-MAKER was not wrong about the patient whom she said was escaping. I just heard the nurses talking about it. I did not say a word about the fact the Medicine-maker told it yesterday, when it was happening. But I was so dumb I thought she was having a delusion. Never again will I make that sort of an error. I must be getting better; more like the doctors and nurses—and they are sane, so they do not believe anything we say.

But the Medicine-maker was right; she was not having a delusion.

There was a class of students being piloted through the "Best" wards yesterday. Thank goodness—whatever else we may have to put up with down here in the hydro, we do not have to prepare ourselves for decorous exhibition everytime a voice bawls, "Visitors on the ward."

But this patient upstairs utilized a group of them to cover her departure. When they were ready to leave she mingled with them. There was no one at the door to check over the number, and when it was opened, she filed out with them. They were a class here from some school. They had come in a truck so she just stayed along with them and when they loaded she piled in and went along.

I do not know how far along on the road they were when

they noted her presence, but I imagine it must have been hilariously funny when they discovered one of the people they had come to see, among them.

She was gone all night and was just returned this morning. I know I do not envy the prospects ahead of her—but I still think I would have enjoyed being among that truck load of students when her presence was noticed!

O, these people who come to look at us—and go through the best wards with their eyes bulging expectantly. They are never allowed down here. They would not be safe. If they were allowed to go through down here some one would have the courage or the lack of control to do what all patients want to do every time they hear "Visitors on the ward."—Visitors on the ward!— If they want to see things in cages—why don't they go to the zoo!

How wide their eyes are with expectancy! And how disappointed they are when they see no indications of the things they came here to see in the people before them. When we become deranged enough to make interesting seeing for the morbidly curious, we are mercifully removed from their view and shut up here in the hydro or taken over to "Three Building."

No, the visiting public does not get a chance to see the people they want to look at. Upstairs on the "Best" ward are many patients far saner than those whose insanity has not been found out. Down here are the kind and type of sights they want to see, yet never do.

No outsider ever sees the inside of the hydro. Even our own families are not allowed to visit us in the hydro. We are taken up to the reception room and if a patient is unable to sit up, they are carried up to one of the wards and put to bed before their company is allowed to see them. Outsiders do not see the hydro. And I can leave them to their fate forever, and hope that in their re-incarnation, they will be small mangy monkeys shut up in a third rate zoo.

The Medicine-maker was turned loose this morning and is sitting in the day-hall in brooding silence. It is the first time she has been out of a strait-jacket for weeks and weeks, but she walks steadily and does not seem weakened by the long confinement. Long months inside have bleached the swarthy texture of her skin to a soft glowing olive color.

She is such a handsome woman—with a compelling fascination which cannot be called "charm" in the accepted sense of the word; nor beauty; nor are any of the other adjectives applicable to her.

She is in a class by herself. In all the world, I do not suppose there is another creature like her. A close-knit, powerful frame, whose contour is that of a woman, but there is something beneath the smooth olive skin suggesting the strength of a gladiator.

It lies along the smooth muscled fore-arm exposed in the short sleeve of the dress she wears; and in the strong tendons of her shapely hands; bleached by many long weeks in the canvas sleeves of a strait-jacket. It is in the long sweep of jaw bone and the strong teeth, whose shape and perfection is suggestive of the teeth of a carnivorous animal; and when her lips draw to a livid line around them the suggestion gives place to—similarity. Above her indescribable eyes are two swooping arches, penciled in one broad flowing line. Above them her hair sweeps backward, so black and bristling it crackles with electric vitality.

To-day is Sunday. There is an unusual bustle of preparation for the Superintendent's round. He will come through shortly and be in such a hurry he will take no notice of the things that have been done to prepare the place for his seeing. His trip is such a whirl of motion his coat tails stream out behind him. But his eyes project shifting penetrating beams of observation. I am sure if anything were not as it should be he would see it instantly; while the things that are as they should be are passed by without seeming recognition.

It is an uncomfortable sensation to feel the eyes of another fall against you for a moment and then pass on to other things; while the lips of the one whose eyes swept you are still turned in your direction to speak a word of greeting; and the whole thing done in such a flash of motion the coat tails did not have time to settle. For this man has a movement swifter than the force of gravity.

Even if you know you have been here for weeks and weeks and never have been seen at all; still it is reassuring to know his eyes have taken in the conditions about you. Yes, it is reassuring to know his hawk-like eyes are watching each detail in the institution.

He inspires such awe in the nurses it emanates from them and settles upon us—and we feel it. No matter how disturbed a patient is, nor how much raving they have been doing; it is a fact that unless they are completely unconscious there are a few minutes each Sunday when they manage to control their raving, and silence reigns; even in the hydro. Whether it is the force of the man, or the importance of his office dominating us; I do not know.

We are in a state of existence that is neither death nor living. It is Madness; and is much more mysterious than either of the other universal experiences attendant upon life. We are the living dead; who have ascended, or descended (according to one's view-point) into this strange limbo of irresponsibility, where we live and pursue our destinies in the strange atmosphere of an insane asylum. Because I am one of the number I feel a kinship with these others binding me closer than those who care for us can imagine. Nor am I alone in feeling it.

The others here have given me in full measure a sympathy and understanding so subtle that those who control us have no idea it flows between us. They think we are indifferent and unseeing, and concerned only with the pursuit of our own whims and fancies; but between these odd people is a system of communication not dependent upon words to make itself felt.

The government here is a vestpocket edition of an old feudal duchy. If we have the colossal impertinence to presume to think for ourselves we get painfully bumped in the transaction. We have been adjudged insane. There is nothing for us to do but go ahead and live up to it; or down to it; as the case may be.

The patients (who are only nuts)—are the serfs in this strange system; immediately over them are the nurses—(and we must call them nurses)—women who do not know how to change the bed of a sick patient—who do not know that lysol must be diluted before it is used. Nurses. One of them was so unthinking she gave a dying woman Apomorphine, which is a sick hypo, instead of a strychnine hypodermic which the doctor had ordered to stimulate her fluttering heart—(and then did not have the moral courage to report her mistake to the doctor).

Later she had no more principle than to laugh about her cleverness in getting away with the lies she told when it was found out. She saw nothing but humor in a dying woman retching with the awful nausea of a sick hypo; (the woman was only a nut; and did not matter).

Nurses. Bah! Nut-herds!

But I have Shakespeare—Thank God for Shakespeare. Take

it away Shakespeare, take it away! I am beginning to get hot under the collar and that is—senseless.

Hey Nonnie—Nonnie. (We add a coupla hot chas, Shakespeare).

See yon beauteous maiden standing singing!—(Stark naked by gravy!—You would see her first!)

Feel the fierce clamor in her soul as it rolls into the world in a mysterious melody of Madness!—(Hells bells, Shakespeare —I'd say she was just another nut—howling.)

See the translucent loveliness that lingers in the litheness of her limbs! I'd say legs, Shakespeare; I'd say that they were very pretty legs and would not go to the trouble of all those alliterations.

But take it and go with it; only do not make me look at her; I feel the nerves along my arms drawing into goose-bumps; the hair on my head rising on end; the nerves along my spine huddling together for companionship; and if she does not quiet down pretty soon, I'll be howling with her.

But here comes the Mother down the aisle, led by two nurses. Her hair is on end too; "starts and stands apart" as Hamlet's stood, if I quote you right. What? You too, can see nothing but the pendulous bulge of her abdomen, hanging, heavy and broken from many births? The trailing bed-ticking straps of her strait-jacket; the swollen lips, trying to shape words she cannot remember? She shapes them into a call for one of her children; the name comes out thickly. She cannot remember what she must make herself say; she has forgotten everything except that something terrible has happened to her and she must call her children to save her.

Her buckling spine will not support her and she falls heavily against the jacket holding her. Now her knees give away so she almost slips out of the jacket. Now the nurses take her arms and propel her along between them but her feet have forgotten the mechanics of walking, one of them is dragging along the floor, bent and turned in at the ankle.

She has just had a spinal "puncture"—which is something done in the treatment of syphilis.

Shakespeare; I tell you I cannot stand it! What the devil is there to write about except to say over and over!

The nuts are all raving—the nuts are all raving—Raving and Dying—and that this is the bug-house—this is the bug-house—Hooray for the bug-house! Fifteen rahs for the bug-house! I'll tell the world it's raw. Not even half baked; just Raw! Plumb—completely—entirely—eternally—everlastingly—irrevocably—irretrievably—undeniably—Raw! Stripped down—skinned off—bleedingly—raw. So raw it hurts terribly. Naked. Uncovered. Stark. Squirming. A fish-worm on a hook. The whole place is heaving and pitching. There is no escaping it—and Hell will be easy after this.

Shakespeare—I am stark mad myself—and I cannot stand it!

There is the "Preacher"—I haven't said a word about the Preacher. Except for my mirror, she is the one who gave me my first sight of an insane person. She was the ugliest thing I ever saw and her insanity has not improved her looks, though it is odd what association with a person will do to the way you feel about them. And it is still more odd, the kinship with them from knowing yourself to be one of them.

They brought her to this grim mausoleum on one of the last days preceding spring-time; when nature was holding a dismal wake over the cold, lifeless body of winter.

I am sure those who brought her felt the grim resemblance the long trip down here bore to a funeral train; and that those who loved her would have felt less grief at bearing all that remained of her to some quiet cemetery where the interment would have ended with the quiet finality of soft earth falling on a silent coffin.

But life was not so kindly disposed toward them; and they brought their loved one; a maniac, raving; to this grim limbo of the living dead. She has expended almost all of life she had in raving; and has portrayed before us a real life drama—so grim and gripping the senses reel from seeing it.

She is locked now in the side room—but the massive door which shuts her away, alone with Madness, is not thick enough to shut out the sound of her raving. It is only a flimsy breakwater; and the noise pours through upon us a swirling torrent. Bones is shrieking; the Pagan is howling; the Camel is singing— Claw-belly is cursing—the Field-mouse is grieving—the little Sick Girl is raving and cursing—and dying—the Medicine-maker is staring, somberly—and as I write it, she threw her head back— and laughed—Laughed, and there is no humor, for her face muscles pulled her features aside to show something better unseen—And I, Shakespeare and I are trying our damnedest to hang on to a pencil. But the doors of "Three Building" are yawning wide for us. And I am a fool to have thought I might build a ladder of words—strong enough—and long enough, to reach out of this.

But the Preacher; let me try to get the Preacher onto paper, before I become a human phonograph and grind out an interminable record; and reproduce an exact duplication, the sound of her raving.

I was still up on the "Best" ward when the Preacher was brought here. Upstairs and in bed with my eternal neuritis, which the Doctor thinks is only hysteria; and he may be right.

But the world has not yet scratched the surface of the capabilities of the human mind, if it is able to create such a convincing pain as neuritis, when it runs amuck and gets tangled up with itself. If the mind can do that much when it is down—there should be no end of things possible if it could be taught how to walk without falling over itself.

The very name "Neuritis" is only another sample of the obsession of these modern doctors, so inflated with sophistication they have transformed whole forests into wood-pulp to make dictionaries of the classifications of diseases—both of mind and body. Not so long ago the malady would have been recognized and treated as a common garden variety of "rheumatiz."

But hysteria, neuritis, "rheumatiz"—or just plain imagination; I was in bed with it, and those in charge recognized the potency of my imagination enough to allow me a hot-water bottle to nurse along with the pain.

Then the Preacher came. The noise of her arrival reached from the street up through the fog into the ward on the third floor and all the patients there flocked to the windows.

I heard the commotion and saw the interest of the others—and my curiosity got the better of my "imagination"—so leaving my hot-water baby, I went to see, too. Down on the street a car had drawn to a stop before the entrance. Three men were struggling with some one in the back seat, trying to drag her out; someone who did not want to be dragged out. A chain holding her was being threshed about, and fell with a clank as her flailing arms flung it aside.

At last they got her out. She was dressed in a short muslin nightgown, big splay feet bare against the wet pavement—and hair escaped from two stringy braids rolled into mats about her head. Her arms still flailed wildly and her voice carried upward, bellowing hoarsely.

A nurse stepped up and threw a blanket about her; something in the gesture and the way she did it was a revelation. I began to have a new respect for these people who give themselves to our care—for there before me was a miracle in the art of managing people. The nurse put an arm about her and marched her inside; and she came. One frail woman doing what three strong men, and chains, had not been able to do.

Another nurse was waiting at the door and together they brought her up the long flight of stairs. She came raving—her voice one long unceasing bellow in which no word was intelligible. Just a steady roaring sound—and when the ward door was opened it burst in upon us like a cataract. It took both nurses and all the patients who could get into the bath-room to bathe her.

A bath is the first requisite for all incoming patients. They are ushered in, thoroughly laundered and put to bed. Sometimes one bath is not sufficient. I have known of two who had to have three tubs of water before they arrived at an allowable state of cleanliness. One old woman went into the bath-room looking like a fullblood Creek Indian; and came out, a snowy-haired old Saint. But they were glad enough to stop at one bath for the Preacher.

They put her to bed, but she would not stay. They gave her a drug, but it was like so much water in her veins. She raved and charged all night and was finally locked up in one of the side rooms.

Next morning she was brought out and put to bed in the dormitory again. The rest of the ward went down to breakfast, leaving she and I alone together. The other nurse was across the day hall in the linen room. I was not afraid of her, but did have a burning curiosity about her, since she was by far the most insane person I had seen up to that time. (Since then, I have had my curiosity about insanity satisfied to satiety—to nausea—to revulsion—and finally—to escape it—I embraced it.)

Presently she arose from her bed and came toward me. I had no idea what was in her mind, but was curious and wanted to know. She was the most unprepossessing proposition that ever approached me. She had never been a pretty woman—and Madness made the very most of her ugliness.

Her skin was weather-beaten and swarthy; her mouth, a great outward bulge of two coarse lips, filled with a whole set of gold crown work, poorly done and covering huge buck teeth. The outer rim of her nostrils was broad and flaring; the bridge somewhat flattened. As I lay in bed looking at her, the flaring flange of her nostrils was suggestive of the mouths of twin storm sewers—huge, black and cavernous. Around them glared her eyes, narrow, blood-shot slits, like two pickled beets in a bowl of clabber. Above them her forehead retreated suddenly into tangled hair at the uneven hairline. Down both cheeks was a broad, deep furrow which piled the flesh on either side into uneven ridges. Her whole face suggested a barren stretch of landscape, filled with hills, ridges, ravines, gullies, and storm sewers. Her baying voice was a human fog-horn.

She thought I was one of her children. To hear a fog-horn talk baby talk is an odd experience. She leaned down, kissed me and told me to move over so she could get in bed with me. I moved to oblige her and threw the covers back, but something in the length of trunk and limb she saw convinced her I was an imposter, not her baby.

She fixed her glaring eyes upon me and I felt a chill run up and down my spine. I also felt something of the stark mad wickedness behind that glare.

"Goddam you! I'm going to kill you, that's what I'm going to do!"

She looked like she meant it.

While I had been willing enough to let her get into bed with me it did not suit my plans to be throttled by a maniac. The hot water bottle was still on my neck. As she jerked it off and hurled it the length of the dormitory, the sudden wrench of pain was the last thing needed to convince me that I should postpone my curiosity till a more auspicious season—so I forgot it, and the pain with it, sprang out of bed and caught both her arms, twisting them behind her.

She glared around at me again—"Did you hear me? I'm going to kill you!"

"You just think you are—you're going back to your own bed quicker than you ever did anything in your life!"

I meant it; she went—because I put her there. The floors up there are polished to a skating rink slipperiness—and her stiffened knees made her slither across them like an ice boat with my propelling knee behind her.

By the time she had reached the bed, I had changed in her mind from her baby to her mother. The illusion was completed when I pitched her into bed bodily and told her I would spank her soundly if she came my way again. She snuggled down in sniffling obedience. The nurse came back in time to hear me make the threat.

She looked at me pityingly and said, "Don't you know she's too crazy to know anything? Go get a jacket and we'll tie her!"

But whether the nurse had under-rated my ability to make an impression or the other woman's ability to retain one, I do not know. But when I was sent to the hydro about six weeks later, the Preacher stopped her raving and eyed me wonderingly.

"What's your name?"

I told her and her face screwed up in puzzlement.

Then she remembered. "Oh sure! Now I remember! You are the woman who put me to bed! Sure—I remember you; you put me to bed. I stayed too, didn't I? You are my friend!"

She has twice been to the hospital, nearly dead from exhaustion and raving. They transferred her the second time on the morning I was sent down here—but she has a vitality that surpasses anything imaginable. Her lungs must be great puffing bellows made of toughest leather. Her voice goes on and on, hours, days, weeks, never stopping. All the drugs they dare give do not quiet her more than a few minutes at a time.

After she returned from her second trip to the hospital and was able to take a few staggering steps, she called me to her. Her brain seemed to clear a little as she asked me where she was and what day it was.

Before I could answer her she interrupted with,

"O, I know where I am! I remember that someone said that I would have to be sent to the insane asylum! So that's where I am! But what day was that? It was Tuesday, wasn't it? and this is Friday."

"Where is my husband and the baby? Are they still waiting here for me? My God! I must go feed that baby; he will be starved to death! Three days! His daddy won't know what to feed him. Who do you see to get out of this place? I've been gone three days and that baby will be starving."

Three days—and it was nearer three months! I tried to tell her she had been very sick and delirious; that the time had slipped up on her. Her distress was so pitiful, she was so bewildered, and because I know the lost feeling that follows raving, I led her to a window to let her see the world outside. Then she might know she had not died and was not facing the unknown conditions after death. But it was the wrong thing to do; the shocks of reality were coming too rapidly for her to adjust herself. She looked out and saw the advance spring had made in "three days." She could not comprehend it and a wild fear for her baby clutched at her.

She turned and almost overbalanced me as she caught my shoulder.

"Listen here; you're my friend, I know you are. You've got to help me get out of here and get to my baby; they will kill him! What do those kids and their daddy know about taking care of a baby! I tell you, they will kill him! You've got to help me get out of here!"

I tried to tell her they would care for him, or that somebody would; that she would have to stay here long enough to gain strength—and pointed out she could not even walk without help, so even if she were at home someone would have to care for her as well as the baby. That she should stay where she was until she regained strength enough not to be a burden upon them. (It was the old, old precedent of evading the issue.)

"But he is a breast baby—I could nurse him, anyway."

Investigating fingers explored the region of her bosom and her eyes dilated with new understanding.

"My God!" she screamed, "I have no milk! My breasts are as dry as a bone!"

The nurses came then and put her again into a jacket.

Her people have come once to see her. I was given the job of getting her up to the ward to receive them. She was almost more than I could manage. She knew she was going upstairs to see her family; her dragging feet could not keep step with the racing eagerness of her mind as she swayed and staggered and lurched heavily this way and that. One minute her weight would all fall against me and the next in some other direction so with each step we were in danger of losing our footing and hurtling to the bottom of the concrete steps.

At last we arrived without serious mishap on the top floor ward. She was put to bed to receive her company while I returned to the hydro.

When her people were ready to leave she would not let them go, so the nurse phoned to the hydro for help. I was dispatched to bring her back. I could hear the commotion from the stairs when the door into the ward was unlocked.

Two little boys were standing in the hall gazing in wide-eyed bewilderment and fright at the strange woman whom they had called "Mamma."

The room was in disorder; a chair was overturned amidst other signs of a struggle. She had both arms about her husband in a straining grip and was pleading frantically with him and reproaching him because he had not brought the baby. I went in and loosened her arms from him, while he stood as someone in a daze. Her face was blazing wild; his, drawn and haggard.

I held her from him but her arms were reaching and clutching while she pled piteously for the baby. He made no move to go, just stood as someone who had lost all power of speech or movement. The children stood watching like statues; white faced and staring. I felt the drama of their lives surging and beating about me; felt my own hysteria mounting, from feeling it. No one came to relieve the tension and I could feel it tightening till it seemed about to strangle all of us. Some one had to do something to break it. I said something to the effect that he could go now as I would take care of her.

The sound of a strange voice seemed to jerk him up.

"Sure. Yes. Of course. Thanks," he said, and went out.

There was something in the look he gave as his eyes passed mine that ought never be seen by anyone but God. The tired slump of his shoulders under his working-man's coat, was more suggestive of pathos than an ocean of tears.

After waiting for them to get down the stairs, I started back with her; the trip still seems like a nightmare. She has seldom been out of a strait-jacket since.

They had brought a great arm load of outdoor grown roses which we put into a syrup bucket on the serving table. She noticed them several times and admired them—but she could not remember they were hers. The idea stuck though, that she had gone up-stairs and had seen her husband and two of her children. She remembers coming down without them—so she thinks they are still up there.

Whenever she is loose she goes staggering and falling toward the door trying to go to them. She wants to see the baby and worries incessantly about him. She has forgotten her breasts are dry and thinks she must go nurse him. She fights when we take her away from the door and calls piteously for her husband to bring the baby to her. Pretty soon it will all be to do over again; no amount of explaining will rid her of the idea they are up there.

She singles me out as the person with the most power to help her. Sometimes I feel I am going madder than the hatter when she fixes me with pain-filled and pleading eyes and begs me—sometimes even on her knees, to allow her to go to her baby.

Or if I will not let her go; to "please, please go and bring him down here. He is hungry and crying; I can hear him crying. I can hear him upstairs crying because he is hungry."

And the tragedy is, that it is real to her. She reminds me over and over that I am her friend; and it is maddening.

She thinks she is called to preach and would be very happy delivering unending sermons to us—if she could not hear her baby, wailing with hunger. She really does have a magnificent voice, deep, resonant and penetrating. But when she is not using it preaching, she lays and calls for hours and hours for her husband to bring the baby down to her.

I have noticed with nearly all these people, when they start raving a certain phrase or pattern of words will be said over and over until it becomes so set in their minds they continue a rhythmic repetition of it, long after every other mental function seems to have ceased. It is like a pendulum set going in their minds, stopping only when the body is too exhausted to further register its swing. One night this woman lay for seven long hours by the nurse's watch and called in a "deep-mouthed bay,"

"Come on down—come on down—come on down—come on down."—She made two syllables of the "down" which made it, "Come on da-own." Never once did she vary the inflection or rhythm or tempo.

It went on and on and on—like the steady beat of a tom-tom, until the very air seemed to have the pattern of the vibration graven into it. There was something lethal and hypnotic about it. I could feel the sound of it graving into my own brain and the rhythm of it beating against my own consciousness until I really believe I must have been half hypnotized.

It was probably a fault in my own nervous system that made me as sensitive to it as I was—but I think, after that experience,

I understand why primitive peoples all employ some form of the tom-tom in worship and in warfare, and at other times when they feel the need of arousing something in themselves beside common-place reactions toward ordinary things.

CHAPTER *8*

THE DOCTOR WAS through again just now—and has re-
deemed himself forever in my eyes from the smug complacency
I accused him of. I saw him stand for a long time by the bed of
the little sick girl, looking down upon the pitiful life within her
as it beats itself out.

He saw her as a human being sees, not as some superior creature who could look on death and madness and be untouched
by it, because he was armoured in a clanking suit of technical
terms.

His armour slipped from him this morning; and he saw her.
Saw and felt the stark tragedy and pain and death, that he with
all his learning is helpless to avert. He saw it with the helpless
eyes of a human who knows he is helpless. His lips were grim
and drawn and there was actual pain within his eyes. Because
I was the next human being whom his eyes fell upon, he did
not remember in time to check himself before he spoke out suddenly in a spontaneous human gesture.

His armour had slipped, he was no longer a being removed
and separated and superior. He was only a helpless human
creature who had seen something the very sight of which could
not be borne alone—but must be fled from and shared with
someone—quickly. Nor shall I ever again resent the fact they

incase themselves in armour—of whatever sort is necessary; for I saw his pain this morning at seeing Madness—nakedly.

I saw the grim line of his lips as he stood looking down upon her—and she was something more than a thing in a test-tube.

I felt the bleak pain in his eyes as he contemplated her recognizing his own helplessness to salvage anything out of the prodigal waste of a human soul born under a cloud—half-doomed before she was formed. For there she lies—dying—before she has lived. Yet in the short span of her life, she has experienced much which is worse than death—in hours of raving, she has lived through whole life-times of pain.

The nakedness, intensity and the shrillness of the things she felt, have finally burned her life to a flickering ember.

In the last day or two she has been quieter because the life is so nearly burned out of her body it can no longer give expression to the Madness driving her.

Death has had his hand on her for several weeks—but she does not know she is dying—and if she did know, she would not stop trying for one minute to find some sort of expression for the Madness consuming her.

Now she is vomiting—her poor sick eyes, blood-shot and swimming. Now her nervous fingers are plucking and picking at the edge of her sheet. Now her hands are fists, drumming a tattoo against the edge of the bed, where they are tied with old stockings. She is flinging herself about in a wild frenzy of restlessness and the sheet, tied corner-wise across her to restrain her, has slipped down, so her young breasts are revealed, beautifully formed, rounded and firm in spite of her long wasting sickness.

Because she is so small and so frail and so helpless—it is maddening to see all of life that she has, in mind and in soul and in body, crunched out and destroyed in such a cruel manner. A monster who stops now and then in his eating to lick slavering chops; from whose teeth are hanging the raw bleeding fibres of live nerves torn from her living body, to be mangled and masticated slowly between jaws dripping red with insatiable cruelty.

The death she dies is too maddening for contemplation; too horrible; and when it comes it will fall as a period to a life which is unthinkable. Life, Death and Madness have contended together over her destiny for twenty-one years—and none of them have had the kindness to close the chapter quickly.

Just yesterday morning I bathed her, as I lifted her frail, wasted body into the great bathtub, she laughed when she felt the water against her and splashed about in it as a pleased baby does. The laughter died in her throat—and the small palm, extended for splashing, convulsed itself suddenly into a fist, and her voice shrieked out shrilly, vile and obscene words filled with hatred and murder. Then her voice became low and soft and full-throated and fell caressingly around the memory of someone whom she had loved.

When I carried her back to her bed her arms caught about my neck tightly in a frenzy of fear, so real and gripping that I had to unclasp them by force.

She looked up at me, crying piteously; then shrieked out in her fright and cowered, trembling, hiding her face in her arms trying to shut out the frightening vision. And though I worked with her calmly and tied her back down in a most matter-of-fact manner; my own soul seethed within me from the madness of seeing her.

I was face to face with the grim recognition that I was helpless to help her—and something within me congealed my boiling rebellion into cold lumps of acceptance.

I cannot accept it—I cannot! Now she is rolling her eyes, cursing wildly. Now she is screaming—her mouth open and straining, her arched back rigid and her eyes dilated with unthinkable horror.

If just one of our law-makers could see her—he could convince the whole body they should lay aside their compunction, indecision and vacillation and pass laws to rigidly enforce sterilization. True—they might make a few errors, but no error of denying the right of procreation to the few whose right to transmit life might be sacrificed unnecessarily, would be sufficient to out-weight the insupportable evidence here in this hydro.—And this is just one "institution."

The world does not have the courage to dispose of such victims in a forthright manner, because it calls itself "Civilized"—therefore it taxes itself beyond measure to keep institutions where they may be hidden from all except doctors and nurses.

The world cannot endure the sight of them—and neither can doctors and nurses. They must either blind themselves with coldness and indifference, or encase themselves in technical armour. If the coldness they train themselves to feel, melts ever so slightly, or if the armour of learning slips from them they turn and flee quickly as all people do when they see something that cannot be borne.

Perhaps my voice is the only one among the great number who have been adjudged insane, with the courage to voice an appeal (only I cannot voice it either—for I am already locked away with those whose voices can never be heard by anyone). But I do wish that I had the power to lift my voice and shout loudly enough to make those on the sane side of living pay some attention—so those whose minds are sane enough to think on the problem might do something about it—something to try to put a stop to this inhuman torture.

Please—Please have the courage to do something about it.

If there is no chance of freeing us, once the snare of Madness has caught us—and if the trap is sprung most often along the path of heredity; please try to decide who is fit to bequeath the heritage of life to an off-spring—and dam up the life streams of the others.

Please give the half-damned ones their freedom. The freedom of never being born! For it is better that life have no beginning than that it be ushered in and gambled against such an ending.

But once they are born, there is that in our thinking which recoils from the heathen custom of strangling—and as we have no sacred rivers to throw our poorly born babies into they grow and mature and perhaps beget others also. Then the largest institutions in the land are given over to the care of those who came out of the shambles.

Creatures who are faced, even before they are formed, with the possibility of being a burden to others—and an unspeakable torture to themselves!

In this "land of the free" and "the home of the brave," ever boasting the slogan that all men are born equal, and by the very fact that they are born are endowed with the inalienable right to life, liberty and the pursuit of happiness—a population is allowed to increase which is in greater bondage than the slaves of the south. For no legislative act: no warfare having to do with martial music and flashing bayonets, can strike off the fetters of Madness.

But the people who are the least fit for the office of parenthood, do not question the moral right of themselves to have off-spring, so long as they have the physical ability. And no one

/127/

else feels sure enough of themselves in the matter to question —lest they interfere with the operation of personal liberty. But anyone who could see what it means to be mad; could see the horrible thing life can resolve itself into for some of its creatures—could not help but think, and then wonder if such creatures as are here in the hydro are not due some consideration and forethought from those sane enough to think for them.

They cannot be freed, once they are bound—and their bondage is a type of slavery and suffering the sane world cannot endure to look upon—and keep its sanity.

If the world is too civilized to put the victims of Madness to death—and so give them freedom—how long, O God—how long will it be before the state will become civilized enough to give them the freedom of never being born!

For there is not one of these people who would make any protest, or voice an objection—if the state had decided they should not have been born. There are even those here who would not draw back greatly; and some would not draw back at all; if the state should pass judgment and say their life were better destroyed. There are some who would welcome the sentence.

But what do my thoughts on the subject amount to? Nothing; exactly nothing. I am one of the number who cannot think straight, and all freedom is denied me because I am insane.

My only expression is to do as these others do; rave out my rebellion here in a mad-house. But surely—anyone who had the courage to look at the wrecks here in the hydro, could not help admitting it were better that life had not found its way to such creatures.

But the world cannot endure that type of seeing—therefore it shuts the victims of Madness away in concealment from all eyes but the doctors and nurses!

Then it sits smugly down and calls itself "Civilized"—and thinks it has lived up to its vaunted claim of civilization when it makes appropriations for our upkeep. I say "the ancient races who stoned us to death showed greater kindness."

No one has the courage to interfere with the actions of God —and whoever suggests it stirs up such a mares-nest that a cry of dissension is heard in all directions. The precious "liberty" of each individual is a thing holy—inviolate—and must not be tampered with.

But where is our liberty—our voice in the matter? Where is our representation—our choice—our chance to be heard. We who are mad—and the thousands now waiting upon the threshold of conception, who will be ushered into the world to fill the insatiable maw of dementia. The state shuts the door on undesirable aliens but the people here are not aliens. They are born of American parents; parents unfit to transmit sane minds and sound bodies but because they are protected by the code of personal freedom, whose right is not questioned.

Three days spent in the hydro would convince any legislature they could vest in themselves a code of enforcement as strict as the "Divine right of Kings." Should they happen in when a young girl is dying—horribly—because she had the poor judgment to be born of a syphilitic mother—they would go back to their lawmaking and put teeth, steel teeth, in the laws demanding sterilization.

Even as I write this there is a stream of profanities and obscenities pouring out of the little sick girl's mouth—so vile, so foul, the very air is crawling and stinking. Her voice does not have the feminine sound of a girl's voice—it is heavy and throaty.

/129/

There is a passion, a vitality—a madness in her speech that makes the words she uses seem pitifully inadequate to express her delusions.

She does not know death is upon her—nor would she care if she did know. Madness is upon her like travail upon a woman with child. It has come. It has claimed her. She can neither avoid it nor satisfy it. It is wasting all the life within her in a prodigal holocaust of raving; is preparing other victims for itself by consuming her here in the presence of all. Death is preferable. Thank God it is coming!

Even the doctor, who is armed with experience and wisdom —turned and fled from the sight of her—and his eyes held the stark look of human pain in them. He felt the grim helplessness, the painful inadequacy of his profession, which has only been able to provide a long name for her Madness. That was not an adequate armour this morning.

There is nothing to be done about it. It is just one of the things that—Is. It is a thing bitter, hopeless and senseless. Much better to dismiss it with a shrug, an up-lifted eye-brow—or by tapping the forehead. After all—she is only a nut. She has no rights in the world. Only a colossal misfortune.

It is only right she should pay a penalty for her poor judgment. The state already has enough on its hands guaranteeing to the parents who bore her—their inalienable right to beget others too.

If babies have no more sense than to be born of such parents, let them pay for their folly. The state cannot be bothered, it has already demonstrated its civilization.

It has set aside huge sums of money to equip nice institutions where they can be sent. There every possible thing is done to prolong the horrible death awaiting them. For the world is civilized. It would be incompatible to resort to the barbarous practices of ending such pain suddenly and mercifully by stoning. Nor can it interfere with a clear conscience—and insist on the right to choose parents less likely to breed such fore-doomed offspring. It might interfere with someone's inalienable liberty.

CHAPTER *9*

THE PLACE IS in an uproar again as it always gets toward night-fall.

Two noisy patients at the end of the room are engaged in an animated conversation. Both are laughing and talking, lying on their beds and facing each other so they talk into each other's eyes. But their conversation is not motivated by a common interest in a single subject; they both talk at the same time—and each is discussing a different subject.

A third one joins in their conversation—and brings a third subject. Another patient is singing—now she has stopped and has commenced to bray like Balaam's ass. Now she is quarreling with the people who inhabit her delusion and the three who were talking are trying harder and harder to convince each other of the things they say.

The nurses will pull the bed of the most animated conversationalist out into the day-hall, where she will continue just as interestedly, whether she has an audience or not. The things these people have to say furnish so much satisfaction in the saying it does not matter whether there is anyone to hear them or not.

All afternoon the Camel has been raving at the top of her voice. Just now her voice is a howl—she thinks it is singing—but it's an ear-splitting racket to the rest of us. She intersperses her singing by fantastic remarks we cannot often catch the meaning of—but when she can make herself lucid enough so we can catch her viewpoint we are convulsed by her humor. She has a slant on things that is ludicrously funny. Now she is spitting on the floor and saying,

"Pheyoo!—Just like old Zeke Turner—the nasty old buzzard! —Shame on me! I shouldn't do it. Remember the Johnstown flood. Shame on me."

But now she is spitting again and rolling her tongue against her uneven teeth like a cat eating cold tallow. Then she is singing again and her voice sounds like a steam caliope—a steam caliope that cannot be directed to make the right tones—but shrieks out in shrill whistles and ear piercing discords.

The Camel has greater lung power than most of the others —and tonight she is far in the lead in the noise-making. The nurse just now came to cover her head with a pillow and is lying across it trying to make her be still. But the sound keeps coming out through the feathers—and though we can hear her, the racket now is little soft puffs and muffled grunts. When the noise gets out into the dormitory it goes running about in little soft peeps—like a baby chick—for it is swaddled in the down of the pillow; so the raucous discord is gone for the moment.

The Camel has more endurance than the nurse, so it is only a little while until the nurse gets tired of her position; the Camel will not give up.

I thought so! The nurse has risen and the Camel has pushed the pillow aside with a forward thrust of her face. Her mouth is spread in a grin stretching widely around her uneven teeth while her tongue protrudes through the gaps where some are missing.

One heavy lid is fallen over one prominent eye. The other is wide open, projecting rays of malevolent delight in the direction of the nurse's retreating back. She is conscious of her triumph and is making more noise than ever.

But her triumph is of short duration, the nurse is coming back with a cup. From the odor curling up out of it as she passed me, I know that the Camel's waking noises will soon be succeeded by her slumbering ones; scarcely less disturbing; she snores like a locomotive. The cup contained "paraldehyde"—Ah! Paraldehyde. Bones calls it "Formaldehyde." The Camel was made to drink it and now she is howling she has been poisoned. But already her howls are beginning to settle into snores—and how she can snore!

She has some interesting variations she will intersperse here and there. The gasoline motor effect, the Hallowe'en noise-maker effect, the put-put-put-put—like intermittent machine-gun fire, as her lips flutter in the gust of her exhaling breath. Then there are other combinations of noises. I know of nothing in this world for a comparison, nor do I know how they are produced. It is all a secret process of her own, but she can turn out some startling effects in plain and fancy snoring.

She is the most ridiculous mortal. There is nowhere in the world another person like her—she is a living, breathing, raving caricature of something a cartoonist dreamed in a night-mare. And no matter what happens the Camel is good for a hearty laugh in the middle of it. She has a long string of euphonious syllables she insists is her name and raises merry cain when any of us do not pronounce the tintinnabulary sequences to her liking. Her voice never loses the caliope effect—even when she cuts down the volume for speaking.

The Camel had only been here a few hours when I was admitted, so we were both new patients up on the "receiving" ward together, and received our "initiation" simultaneously. Then each weighed more than we do now; and it was a stock joke up there about what a formidable looking pair we were. I was laundered and put into a bed next to hers where the nurse could get to us quickly. That was in case we evolved any wild ideas and tried to act upon them.

They allowed us to get up in a day or two, and as our own clothing was still in the marking room, they brought us state garments. Two of the better patients were detailed to bring them in to us and see that we got into them properly.

I drew a little old witch of a woman who had a great hump on her back. She stood holding the garments for me right-side-to, to prevent me donning them wrong-side-out or hind-part-before. Since we had been adjudged insane, our intelligence is reckoned at the start to be no higher than the lowest imbecile. We go on with that rating until we distinguish ourselves sufficiently to gain a higher one—or live down to it and justify the supposition.

The clothing consisted of cotton hose and underthings and brand new dresses of percale print—mine of pink and the Camel's of blue. These latter surprised me; I had taken for granted the "state" clothing would be some drab sort of uniform. Nor were they as ill-fitting as might be supposed. The dresses sent to the hydro are as drab and dirty a grey as could well be imagined—they are used interchangeably for clothing or scrub rags—according to the need which arises first. The dresses for the better wards are given more careful attention; both in material and construction, as well as care. The dresses for the hydro are constructed along the lines known as a "bungalow," which is a strip of material for front and rear, seamed down the sides; slits left for arms and a hole cut through for the head.

But the Camel had not seen the hydro dresses so she had no appreciation of the bright new print brought her. She wanted her own clothing and protested loudly at putting on the other. At last they got her dressed and she set out to hunt her own.

A dozen times that day she sprang up and started out to hunt them. Each time someone would head her off, turn her back to her chair and explain patiently and in detail that her clothes were still in the marking room and she would have to wear "state" ones till they were returned.

At last the idea stuck. She gives voice to her thoughts while they are in process, "State clothes. State clothes. State—clothes. This dress (scrutinizing it) is a 'state dress.' My own nice clothes are gone. Stolen. I must wear 'state' clothes. The state belongs to Governor Murray. The clothes belong to the state. O-O-O-H! Then they are Bill Murray's clothes! This is Bill Murray's dress! My God! And his socks. I thought I recognized the odor! Why, you didn't even wash 'em before you put 'em on me! Take 'em off! Take 'em off! They'll give me the mange! They'll give me the itch. They stink! I can feel fleas crawling in 'em! Let me get out of 'em quick!" And she proceeded to get out of them quickly.

The nurse came running and shook her and glared at her but it was no use.

"Me wear Bill Murray's clothes? That haven't even been washed! I should say not! I am a respectable woman. I never did an undecent act in my life! Do you think you are going to get me to wear those old phooy!, huey!, stinky! things. They haven't even been washed!"

"Alfalfa Bill—he's the guy who started the war with Texas. He sent my son down to the Red River Valley in a uniform, with a gun to fight the Texans if they came across the bridge.

Phooey, Alfalfa Bill, his socks smell like alfalfa, after it's been wet—or after the cows have eaten it. Pheyou, Alfalfa Bill and Huey Long! They both stink—so do their clothes, I'm not going to wear 'em. I'm not going to let any of his old ticks or fleas or itch get onto me. The nasty things; go put 'em back under the rocks where they come from."

At last they convinced her it was those, or none, so she sat in a chair and tried to draw herself into as small a bunch as possible so her protesting epidermis would not touch the offensive garments. She helped the process all she could by catching the garments and stretching them out from her as far as she could. Several times she sprang up and peeled the dress off over her head as though it really was crawling with fleas.

That night she decided she was tired of the bug-house and was going to go places and do things; particularly to the nurse if the latter did not get out of her way and let her go. I was already awake (you do not sleep well the first few nights in an insane asylum) and I distinguished myself spectacularly by coming to the aid of the nurse. We took a sheet from my bed with which to tie the Camel. The next morning when she had to be dressed by force it just seemed to fall easily to my lot to help again with her.

I dressed her feet while she kicked like a Missouri mule and bellowed all sorts of protests. It was Bill Murray's unwashed socks she rebelled at the most. At last she was dressed, even to the "socks." By the time the operation was finished we had all fallen very low in her esteem; were still falling. Governor Bill Murray sinking first in the general precipitation—and fastest, for he had already reached the bottom of her contempt before we started and she had to work very hard to make new depths for him to sink to. She was determined he should occupy the very lowest place in her contempt; so she had to tower to great heights of out-raged dignity to keep her emotional perspective.

Thus she grew and expanded until her hatred became bottomless, with Bill Murray far, far down in its unmeasured depths; and she, "a respectable woman who never did an undecent act in her life," far, far above in the serene atmosphere of her own unquestionable superiority. And because she had been overpowered by brute force and unbelievable indignities had been heaped upon her while she was down and helpless—she was none the less a perfect lady; and would convince the low archconspirators so, by conducting herself as one.

She knew it would be "entirely beyond our poor power of comprehension, because we were all such low, vile, specimens of undecency we had no sensibilities for the appreciation of anything fine."

So she went into the day-hall and seated herself in a rocker, whose strident creak made a fitting accompaniment for her caliope voice as she sang, "In the Sweet Bye and Bye"—rocking dangerously far back and bringing her feet down with a crash to mark the rhythm.

The day nurses coming on duty, heard her more than a block away.

"For goodness sake," one of them asked as she unlocked the stair door and came in, "What's the matter with her?"

To which the night nurse gave over her shoulder as she started down, an answer. Brief—brittle—inclusive.

"For goodness sake—What's she here for?"

So she was sent to the hydro and in due time I followed. She was sleeping heavily under a drug; snoring loudly while I lay in a sopping wet bed enjoying the doubtful comfort and benefit of a "pack."

She woke up about the time I was dressed. She saw me and let out a joyful cry of recognition, calling me over to her bed. She called me "Little-Pink-Dress" and insisted she knew me when I was a "little curly-haired baby"; that my mother was her best friend and she had helped nurse her through her last sickness: that she knew and loved all my people, "knew and loved them, every one," my grand-mother and all my brothers and sisters.

By this time she was crying and asked me through her tears if I were not going to kiss her. Of course I did, for I was touched by her feeling—even though I knew she was all wet and could not possibly have any memory of me except as the person who had held her and put "Alfalfa Bill's unwashed socks" on her.

My mother is still living and my grand-mother died long years before the Camel was born, I am the only living child, so there are no brothers or sisters. The only "curly hair" I ever had was bought at a beauty shop and is now a shaggy and wornout permanent, not too successful to start with. She was surely all wet. Very wet indeed, because the nurse was coming down the aisle at that moment with fresh, dry sheets for her bed.

Several weeks later I was helping the nurses wash the walls at house-cleaning time. We had got around to the side-room; the nurse unlocked the door and we commenced cleaning there. The Camel was its occupant at the time. Usually when a patient is in the side-room, they are in a strait-jacket, but the Camel was not tied down on this occasion. She had been raving and charging about so much she was getting all the others started—for when one starts to rave the others all follow, according to the whim and caprice of each.

She watched us at work and said something about us cleaning so carefully. The nurses and I were both on our knees washing the lower part of the walls—(for Claw-belly had been the previous occupant and she always has a copious and inexhaustible supply of spittle, which she spreads around freely). The Camel was sitting on the edge of the bed with her knees hunched up to make a support for her elbows; her chin was cupped in her hands.

She asked again why we were going to all the trouble of so much cleaning. The nurse told her we were fixing the "bridal chamber" for her particular benefit. Whereupon she began to unfold herself from her hunched position and finally came almost erect. She rose from the bed and began to amble up and down the room. She seemed more like a caricature than ever—with her hands supporting her back because it was about to buckle up beneath the great bulging weight of her shoulders. She had no extra support to give her knees—so they weaved back and forth as she walked, giving her body a swaying motion.

The suggestion of a "bridal chamber" sent a stream of ludicrous associations ambling through her brain. Her voice became more like a caliope than ever as she released her clownish humor into the room—where it trailed along after her and became a whole circus parade for our entertainment.

"Bridal chamber—Bridal chamber—Bridal chamber! Well—Well—Well! So it is to be a 'bridle' next. I knew all along they had some such idea about me! Why already I've been fed more oats than old Beck and Kate have eaten all winter; Beck and Kate are two old mules and I've been enough like their papa, the jack-ass, to wear a horse-jacket all spring. Bill Murray's horse jacket full of fleas and mange and itch!

"I wouldn't mind the fleas so much—if I could catch them. And I don't mind the mange so much—if I could get my hands free to scratch. But that's the trouble in the first place; I couldn't

/141/

get my hands loose long enough to catch the fleas or scratch the itch; they were tied down in the damned old stinkin' horse-jacket. The stink, that's the thing which gets me down altogether! The stink!! It's worse than the fleas I couldn't catch or the mange I couldn't scratch—there's nothing that can be done with such an odor except smell it. And now if you have decided all I need is a 'bridle'—O—what a relief! Bring it along and I will wear it gladly. While you are about it you might as well bring the 'chamber' too, since the two seem to go together and I need something. Unless you let me go out behind the barn—for I need to go somewhere."

We had given up all hope of washing walls and were leaning against them helplessly; we could not have stopped her if we had tried. She could not go "behind the barn" but she did go to the stool-room—and lathered all the soap and Dutch Cleanser she could find, poured a can of coal oil in for good measure, then put it into her hair.

All those things are now locked in the linen-room—before that, the Pagan had eaten half a can of scouring powder and a bar of Saman soap. And I think she is the one who ate most of my pencil.

The Schizo strolled over to me today, looked over my shoulder and asked, "Whatcha writin'?"

"Nothing much," I stated. "Just a lot of tripe, but it helps take the pressure off. It's a sort of safety valve. When I feel madness creeping upon me I grab this pencil and, while I concentrate on it, my mind is relieved. Right now I'm not feeling much of anything. Just passing the time away with a piece of paper." The Doctor says, "Go to it. It won't hurt you, might help; so keep it up."

"Well," said the Schizo, "that's a new one. Does it really help?"

"Sure," I answered, "it's done more for me than all the fancy packs, paraldehyde and psychiatry put together."

"Hm," she mused, "guess I better try that, too. I've tried everything else. Nothing does any real good."

Leaning back from the serving table I asked curiously, "Just why are you here? You're not violent often. You're not wild. You don't 'rave' much and I just plain don't get it."

"Well," she said, "I'll tell you. You look like a good guy, even if you are as big as a bulldozer and as ugly as a mud fence."

"I had two strikes on me from the start," continued Schizo.

"Two strikes?" I questioned, "how do you mean that?"

"I'm a Juke," she answered simply.

"A Juke, what's that? Do you mean if I give you a nickel you'll play?"

"No," she smiled, "it would take more than that; if I were still 'playing.' But," she said vehemently, "do you mean to say you don't know what a 'Juke' is? Good God in Heaven, I thought everybody knew all about them."

"No, I really don't. What is it? I just figured that was the people who made music boxes and such."

She laughed mirthlessly and said: "A 'Juke,' honey, is one of the two thousand and eighty-six descendants of a woman called Margaret, mother of criminals, and her five sisters."

"Never heard of 'em," I stated, "what's this, two thousand and eighty-six criminals?"

"No, not all criminals. Some were just paupers, some were drunkards, some were crooks and one, only one, was a famous man."

"What's this all about?" I queried. "No family is without its share of black sheep."

"Black sheep. You tickle me. Our family was a whole flock of ebony ewes and sooty-looking rams," she said and again gave that mirthless laugh.

"Well, come on, 'give,'" I said. "Let's hear how that put you here. And, by the way, what was the other 'strike'? You mentioned two."

"Oh, skip it," she said, "hellfire, ain't I got enough trouble already without trying to explain to a big, beefy ox what a 'Juke' is? Why don't you read your history or were you so damn busy learning all those quotations from Genesis or Revelations or the Apostles or whatever it is you never learned any history." She walked over to one of the windows and stood there clenching and unclenching her hands, saying to herself:

"Why was I ever born? Why couldn't I have been a descendant of George Washington or Patrick Henry or plain old John Smith? No, I gotta be a 'Juke' and I gotta pay. I shoulda jumped in the river as soon as I found it out. It's a great life if you don't weaken, but who-in-ell can be strong with that kind of blood in their veins?"

There she stayed until time to eat again.

CHAPTER *10*

THE DOCTOR IS in here again to look at the little sick girl. He is giving instructions to the nurse to have her transferred to the Hospital Building. Bones is stalking behind him as he finishes his rounds among the others. Her talon fingers reach for his coat-tail.

He turned and asked: "What do you want?"

Her flapping jaws framed a request to go home.

He refused her abruptly as he turned and went out through the middle door into the day-hall. She has not straightened up yet but is still standing in exactly the same position—and already his key has clicked in the lock on the outside door. She placed her arms sharply akimbo upon her loose hips and I do not know whether it was to the doctor or to the door which clicked behind him, she addressed her fervent, "O you sunuva-bitch!"

The nurse has said that I may go with her when she takes the sick girl to the hospital—(if I will put on a pair of stockings). So whether I am in my right mind or not, I am sitting fully clothed, waiting. You learn a new appreciation for fresh outside air and sunlight when you are confined behind solid oak doors and padlocked windows; so I am anticipating the prospect of a trip through the grounds—though I do wish it were a different sort of an errand.

And now we are back. The stretcher came with six men patients for carriers, in charge of their attendant—though only two of them were needed. Her slight weight added little to the weight of the empty stretcher. She went raving to her death and we shall never again see her. She was small and dear to me for I have often helped care for her. She was so helpless and clung to us with childish fright—no, not childish, but something stark and terrible. Her frail child's body held a soul tormented with an anguish greater than she had sensibilities to cope with. It has burned her life to an ember with the fierceness of its raving. But the day was so very lovely it absorbed the sadness of little humans living in the glory of its radiance. The destiny of people does not matter to the spring-time.

The grounds, well groomed, with growing shrubbery, basked in joyous contentment, spreading their beauty in voluptuous abandon. From the road a garden stretched down through a terrace where a rock wall made a border for the different shades of green things, which were the setting for a great bed of geraniums; whose blossoms glowed and sparkled like a living ruby, set with care and mounted in growing filigree. They flaunted in the sunlight all the triumph of their living; yet did not disclose the secret of how they could, by growing, draw such living riotous color from the dull brown soil holding them.

A small lake down below them caught the clouds floating over, so the narcissi who sought their own reflection could not see plainly. They peered and peeked and nodded and waited with impatience for the clouds to float away. The white breast of a pigeon flashed the sunlight down upon us and wheeled so close above us we could feel the rhythm of its flashing wings in flight.

But the sad little cavalcade bearing a mad girl to her dying, left no sign or trace of passing on the spring-time. The air closing around us did not rustle as we stirred it. The world, which is the setting for all there is of living, is filled with creatures who are unable to share any thought or feeling or know anything of what life means to the others.

And here in the hydro, the naked drama continues, yet it is more mysterious here where all the covering is stripped away. The mystery of it is seen more plainly but there is no key given to understand it. Life speaks a strange language here in the hydro.

Another patient came to take the bed left empty. She, too, will go quickly, unless they can check the fever raging through her. In spite of ice-packs and cloths wrung from cold water the thermometer registers almost one hundred and ten degrees! Death seems to be standing very close to that bed.

There is another drama of more sinister aspect afloat down here. When we returned from the hospital errand, the nurse in charge drew the other into the linen-room. After a few minutes they called me aside and led me in with them. I went wondering; there is no such thing as privacy here.

I could not imagine why I was being called aside secretly. When the door was closed she asked me if I had noticed any one tampering with the two back bathtubs. I had not- and my curiosity overcame the knowledge that "reasons" are not given us, so I asked her "Why?"

She eyed me narrowly—and I felt an accusing suspicion behind her eyes which made me acutely uncomfortable; though I had no idea what was of such import they should be so secret about it. So I waited while she turned over in her mind the advisability of taking me into their confidence. At last she told me.

"Two of those metal rods have been taken off the bathtubs. The doctor missed them. I have hunted everywhere for them while you were gone. But I haven't been able to find them yet. I thought perhaps you might have noticed something."

I did not have an idea to offer.

"It doesn't matter in the least you know, but I would like to find them. Don't say anything to the other patients. Just keep your eyes open."

Although she tried to discount the seriousness of the situation I knew she was uneasy. It does not lend to peace of mind to know that two grim weapons are concealed somewhere among fifteen people, insane enough to do anything. It is the Medicine-maker of whom they are the most fearful, I know their fear is not without foundation. There is something more sinister about her than most of the others. While I have never thought of myself as being a physical coward, I have seen things in her eyes I did not have the courage to look upon. She has been tied down for months and was only just recently let out of a strait-jacket. It does not take any imagination at all to vision some of the things that might happen if she got her hands on those rods. They would be deadly weapons if wielded by her powerful hands in the frenzy of Madness.

But whether it is she or one of the others who took them; whoever it was has certainly done an excellent job of concealing them. This place has been turned up-side down and wrong side out and still they are not located. One of the nurses herded the Medicine-maker into the day-hall. The other nurse and I, under cover of changing mattresses have searched her bed carefully. Then we put her mattress underneath one of the other patients. We have climbed up and dusted all the radiators and shaken all the curtains, so we know they are not hung by a string or a stocking somewhere in the grating. We have moved everything movable. The search was carried on under cover of a general cleaning, but no rods were found. There is nothing which has not been cleaned and dusted, nothing which has not been rearranged, nothing which has not been looked in, on, or under. But where are those rods? Shakespeare; page Sherlock Holmes; we cannot find them!

The nurses talked it over in my presence and have come to the conclusion, since they cannot find the rods, it must be Claw-belly who took them. They pointed out other times and occasions when she has done similar things.

"I know in reason she is the one who took them off. We never let her out of a jacket that she doesn't do something like that! She is just a damned monkey, into everything! But if she did get them off she wouldn't know what to do with them. She is too crazy to think about trying to fight with them. She hasn't got that much sense!"

To which the other answered with a question which I was thinking too.

"But if she did take them, what did she do with them?"

"How should I know? Swallowed them, maybe. We'll watch her stools!"

This was good wit, but poor logic. Even a maniac with a voracious appetite for inedibles, could hardly swallow two solid copper rods eight or ten inches long, two inches thick and nickel plated.

One of the nurses voiced a bitter objection to the senseless idea of having such tubs installed when they are of no more benefit than ordinary bathtubs. Even the stoppers are so big and heavy they must be guarded along with the paring knife and ice pick. From where I sit, I can see the rods left on the other two tubs;

it does not make for greater comfort to know they are curved to fit the hand.

But where are they? Who has them? And what will they do with them?

Those are grim questions becoming all the grimmer against the noise and raving in the background. All these people are violently insane; not responsible for their acts. Those are grim words to use in connection with nickeled copper rods; curved to fit the hand for grasping!

While the twilight deepens on the world outside, in the hydro the noise of raving rises to higher pitches of dementia; as it always does with nightfall. The night nurses are on duty, visibly more nervous than the day crew were. Partly because they are newer at the work but more, because they know it is going to be tough to sit through the long watches of the night and guard fifteen people; at least one of whom is heavy and pregnant with unborn acts of violence and the others entirely capable of them when filled with hatred. The knowledge that somewhere, hidden, are the weapons, waiting, doesn't make them more at ease.

I lie here awake and waiting too; they are people and I am a person who knows what is in the air, and feel a responsibility to keep my faculties alert to help them if necessary. Of course they do not know but what I might have taken them, but I feel something of the confidence they have towards me, in comparison to some of the others; the Medicine-maker in particular. In my hearing, they discussed the possibility of getting an order to put a jacket on her. She has done nothing to deserve one and until she does they cannot tie her. They were bitter against the day nurses for not putting her in one before they left—the day nurses may tie a patient without an order. I have no idea why. It is just another of the odd things that seem to be without logic.

When I first came here I noticed the uneasiness all of them felt toward the Medicine-maker and asked one of them why they were so cautious.

"Oh," she answered lightly, (the woman was tied down). "Don't you know? Her highest ambition is to kill a nurse!"

And tonight the nurse in charge gave voice to bitterness:

"I don't see why they didn't tie her before they left! We can manage the others but she is as strong as an ox! She is just waiting for a chance when we are having all we can do with someone else to jump in and finish one of us! I would not have gone off, and left her untied if they had been coming on duty—and I don't see why they left her loose! But they don't care how hard a time we have, just so they get through okay!"

I felt the grim uneasiness in the tense lines of their shoulders and their swift flashing eyes as they sit together at their table, one of them on either side so they may command a view of the whole hydro. My bed is near them—I am awake and waiting too, and know the day nurse watched when she questioned me; and that there was grim suspicion behind her narrowed eyes. I know I am not free from suspicion. And yet, because I know I am innocent, I have the feeling they should know it too. But someone took those rods. The fact I am awake may make them more uneasy than if I were asleep; their training has taught them they can trust no maniac.

I do have one consolation. I know I shall not have to go through the nightmare of asking for a strait-jacket and being refused. The nurse thought I was calm and composed! She could see no deeper than the shallow exterior and did not know what things were underneath it. She did not know my apparent smooth self control was just a thin layer hiding a volcano. But I knew it; they knew it, too, before the thing was over. The doctor's word is law in an insane asylum. There is no appeal for either the patients or nurses. I can depend upon the fact they will not disobey it.

If he were to tell me to step up and stretch my neck forth on a chopping block I do not suppose I would question his judgment. Though I know of one or two occasions when he has made some pretty bad errors. I suppose everybody is allowed a certain quota of mistakes. Doctors are more fortunate than others and, as some one said, they bury their errors.

There are many things here that breed discontent and resentment, but personally, I don't know how they could be eliminated. It does seem as though everything possible is done to make it harder for us to cooperate; but then we are insane; and are not supposed to be humans. The sooner we learn to accept it the better. It is not such a bad arrangement, once the fact is accepted; there is freedom from trying to live up to any law other than your own whims and notions. The more insane a patient is, the better that individual fares.

Tonight I lie here—waiting; my strength may be needed. It would be a good thing if some of these nurses had a little of the arrogant superiority taken out of them, but not with curved metal rods held in a maniac's hand; they wouldn't have a chance to profit by the experience. Especially if the Medicine-maker has the rods—and uses them. One blow aimed by her powerful arm would end all need for learning anything!

It is odd I should feel so much responsibility for their safety— I am certain my sympathy is more with the patients than the nurses. I have felt my own hands clench into fists more than once at things I have seen them do—but had no way to protest, any objection we voice is "raving." But I am sane enough to know that curved metal rods are not the means of redressing the wrongs done here. Besides that reason, there is one more personal. I am still a fairly "good" patient which means I still make an effort to uphold a system which is ridiculous; and that I secretly abominate.

In other words, I suppose I would even stay awake and alert to help the nurses whom I dislike the most. I am so loyal to my particular "Goddess" that any patient insane enough to attack her will have to account to me personally. And if one should hurt her, it would be a grim accounting. It shall not happen if my strength means anything at all. There are also other patients who would just about mob any one who tried to hurt her. Her kindness to us has purchased the passport for safe conduct when she comes among us.

Though we are insane, and not quite human beings that very fact gives us keener appreciation of the kindnesses shown us; when any are shown us. If a nurse treats us as human beings she gains for herself a devotion dog-like in its unquestioning loyalty. Of course the loyalty and appreciation may be expressed in such an odd manner the one for whom it is meant misses the significance; as for example, right this minute I have the feeling the nurses are more uneasy because I am awake than they would be if I were sleeping; they distrust all of us. And there is nothing anyone of us may do that will eradicate the fact that we are insane, and therefore not to be trusted.

That means there is nothing left for us but to live and act according to whatever mysterious impulses are walled up within our being. We are strange, alien creatures and have little in common with ordinary human beings.

Perhaps I am wrong in my conclusions; too prone to see the

morbid side of things. The nurse just now came to me and touched my shoulder saying that if I would turn my head to the foot of my bed where the light was better, she would bring me a book from the library. I may read! An unheard of concession.

She brought it, saying the one condition was that I should have it beneath my pillow and be "asleep" when the night supervisor made her rounds. I consented gladly; and wandered ecstatically along the "Friendly Road" with David Grayson—which was odd reading for such a setting. The book is poetry; quiet and pastoral. It set rhythm going within me which made me feel I had experienced all that life holds of living. That book brought me all the broad sweep of sunlit meadows plus the peace and quiet of living deeply by the side of dusty highways.

Yet I could not forget the present. The nervous tension of others' restless sleeping and the greater tenseness lurking in the background shadows were the reasons for my reading. The tenseness increased, it gleamed from the concealed reflection of metal weapons waiting the moment to strike out in sudden murder; while over all the two extremes of living, the night spread a blanket of soft-drumming raindrops.

The world has spun around into the morning—and nothing eventful happened through the night. Except I saw another example of the things these nurses labor under. With almost no experience, training or preparation, they are placed over us. The regime they work under is stern and demanding; they are watched almost as closely as we are. Their own pride in their lofty classification as "nurses" prevents them from accepting the help some of us might give them. It is intolerable for them to take suggestions from the inferior people they are placed over. Though there are several of the patients even in the hydro with enough practical experience to change a bed and who know that lysol must be diluted!

Last night as I lay "sleeping," according to instructions, a little incident occurred which was both ludicrous and pathetic. It showed what happens when teachers, waitresses and laundry workers are put into white dresses and called "nurses" before they know what it is all about. These two were changing the Camel's bed. She had been given a purgative—and then paraldehyde. Her bed was in need of changing!

The supervisor caught them in the middle of the unsavory chore. They were going about it in their usual unusual manner. This was to loosen the sheet all around, then catch the corners at the foot—and pull; then put the fresh sheet in under the patient's head and pull again—till it came down far enough beneath the whole length of her body to tuck in at the foot—and never mind the wrinkles! Last night it was nothing short of pitiful. The Camel had provided ample pollution to start with— and they, by their odd method, spread it in every direction, and were themselves splattered with it.

The supervisor caught them when they had the soiled sheet about half off. Their grip on the corners slackened when they felt her unbelieving eyes upon them. Their embarrassment was acute and painful—she had stopped stock still and was staring at them as though she could not believe the tale her eyes told.

In her impatience at their ignorance, she did not consider they had had no chance at training—but repaired that lack immediately by taking them in hand and giving them a lesson in the mechanics of bed-changing; accompanying the instruction with a sarcasm more fitting had they been afforded a previous chance at learning. It was a fitting rebuke for their smug self-satisfaction at their own intelligence. If they had never even seen a sick-bed it does seem they could have devised a more intelligent way to change one. But here they are thrown only with those whom they credit with having no sense at all. That very fact petrifies their own intelligence. They become hopeless bigots and learn nothing until they ram their heads against the criticism of their superiors.

CHAPTER *11*

THE NURSES HAVE not stopped in their search for the missing pieces of metal—but so far they have found no trace of them. They still think it was Claw-belly who took them and that she either slipped them into the bundle of soiled linen waiting to go to the laundry or dropped them down the wide mouth of the drain pipe. They have probed into the pipes with a wire but couldn't tell whether or not they were obstructed. At any rate they have decided there is no possible hiding place which has not been investigated.

But if Claw-belly took them, she is going to have scant chance of doing anything else for a while; for the nurses are chasing her now with a strait-jacket. They are both after her as she races about like a monkey. The bed-ticking straps of the jacket are trailing and sailing as the nurse who has it runs to the end of the dormitory to head her off—but she saw the intention and dashed to the opposite side. Now she is leaping from bed to bed, catching the shades at the windows and tearing them from the rollers.

The Camel let out an awful bellow when Claw-belly stepped in the middle of her stomach—now she has thrust her face forward to take in the show and is enjoying it hugely, shouting encouragement and directions to first Claw-belly and then to the nurses.

Claw-belly's legs are so long she cleared one bed completely in a spraddling leap. But her foot caught in the fold of a sheet— and now they've caught her.

They are putting her into the jacket, and as usual, she is howling curses at them. Now they have her to the bed and one of them is sitting astride her with a pillow over her face—for also as usual, she tried to spit on them. The other is tying the straps to the bed-rail, but her legs are still flying and kicking so they are tying them too, keeping well out of reach of the showering spittle. Now they have left her and she has gone back to her howling and cursing. The nurse is returning with a sheet to pin into a tent above her.

Bones is at a window calling for "Bill" to come free her. She shouts and shouts and offers "six hundred dollars" to anyone who will come get her out. The convulsive grip of her hands stopped long enough in tearing at her own flesh to catch her gown at the neckband and rip it to the hem. The nurse is shaking her; trying to send her away to the stool-room where she can continue her raving in comparative privacy.

Finally she has the idea they are sending her away—and she shrieks with new terror. But at last she starts and walks through the door with a disjointed motion; her body thrust forward, hanging loosely from the hips. Her shrieking continues from behind the closed door of the stool-room where she is alone with her madness. The nurse is phoning to request a drug for her.

They have brought her outside again and put her on the bed, tying her hands to the rail. She is lying there calling and pleading—her eyes do not look like human eyes; but something not good to see. Now she is calling my name and pleading with me to "save her." But what can I do about it? Nothing, exactly nothing. A drug will stop her pain for a while, perhaps—but it will all be to go through again as soon as she awakens. There is nothing another can do to free a soul stretched on a rack of torture their own mind built for them. It is maddening to see the pain she suffers; and to know there is no help for her. But the drug is taking effect quickly and that is something. Sometimes they are so distraught a drug has no more effect than so much water. Being demented, we are not deluded by "psychological" medicine, as administered by your favorite "bedside manner."

Poor old Bones is such a pathetic creature, yet humor lurks often about her. One time she set up an awful howl for a drug, when another patient was being given one. To hear her beg for it was to be convinced she is a confirmed addict. But she isn't; she just took a notion she wanted a hypodermic because the other woman was being given one. She howled and she begged and at last the nurse phoned an order for it. Before the order could be executed Bones had switched to the other extreme—and when she saw the hypodermic syringe she rebelled against it. She was louder in her objection than when she was pleading for it. It took three of us to hold her still for the nurse to give it. When the needle pierced her thigh she let out such a yell anyone would have thought we were tearing her leg off.

There is a little grey kitten down here—and the next morning poor old Bones went about shrieking and howling and wringing her hands and lamenting, "O, my God, my God! They gave me a hypo last night, they gave me a hypo last night! They gave everybody a hypo last night; Everybody!—Everybody! They even gave one to the cat!"

One dismal day when they had given her a drug the night before she went about wringing her hands and howling they had given it to her under her tongue. It is she who always calls

/159/

paraldehyde, "formaldehyde," and gets all mixed up; going quite into detail about the things done to her in an undertaking establishment! She manages to make it very suggestive and revolting. To see a skeleton stalk about, shrieking; with only a moth-eaten blanket of flapping skin thrown about it—is to have your own mind filled with wonder if maybe it wasn't true!

It is odd what living here with these people does to you. There can be little companionship motivated by any common interest in a specific subject. There is no common meeting ground for conversation or exchange of opinions—and yet, there is something that flows between us, I think, greater and more sympathetic than if we were able to converse intelligently with each other.

We know each other better than most people in other places ever learn to know one another. Our understanding is greater than any explanation that could be contained in words. I do not know what it is, because I have no understanding of it—and yet I have felt it keenly when it was in operation; an invisible current of communication which brought very close to my own soul things others were feeling. And more than once there has been evidence of keen understanding and sympathy in the hearts of these others towards me, flowing out in mysterious channels, so hidden, so subtle as it flowed through the turmoil of their raving that I do not wonder at the fact sane folk miss it completely.

People who are sane know little of the things communicated by other means than the clumsy speech organs. Though there is little communication in the accepted sense of the word between these people here, I think I must be very demented myself for thinking the understanding between us is greater than other people have.

All the small things which are the grip of sanity have fallen away and we are all run together and mingle as one in the great brotherhood of dementia. We share as one person the things each experiences individually. I have looked upon these others in their madness and felt myself slip into it too; felt my own soul crumble and fall apart because I could not escape seeing things better unseen.

All that is Madness—and I sit here and write it—and know that it is very probable I shall wind up on "Three Building."

It was the Farm-woman's sister who first ripped the shielding curtain aside, giving me my first insight into that mysterious means of communication. No words passed her lips. In describing it I cannot do much more than record the things our bodies were engaged in. There are no words with enough significance and meaning to explain the elusive and subtle thing which passed between us.

I did not know at the time she was the Farm-woman's sister. What resemblance there may be lies beneath the exteriors—for they are as unlike as two people could be.

The Farm-woman is impeccably neat about her person and the other is as slovenly and uncaring of her appearance as though she had no consciousness of it at all; and she probably hasn't. Both have smooth olive skin; but the sister's never has a well bathed look and her hair is never combed unless the nurses or someone else insists upon the chore being done. She moves with a listless step in sharp contrast to the energetic walk of the other.

However, it is not the disagreeable things about her that were the basis of the fascination she held for me. If those things are dwelt upon and enlarged, they obstruct all other seeing. She is insane—and since that fact is established her actions and conduct are answerable only to her own weird personality. From the first, there was something fascinating to me about her. It often made me wonder about her and I have sat and watched her while I tried to figure out what made me feel differently toward her than to some of the others.

I was curious about her—and yet it was not all curiosity, some of it perhaps was revulsion, but the answer was not contained in any physical attraction or repulsion but in something more mysterious, something much deeper, something which had to do with that mysterious force called personality, for lack of a better name. There was a still, chiseled—chilled—perhaps stupid, quality of repose about her showing through the placid lines of her features, and even her walk was suggestive of a phrase I remember from childhood, when one child wouldn't give up a swing to another until they let the "Old Cat Die."

Everything about her suggested she was "letting the old cat die," that the life within her was going on of its own volition, that she was not interested in it or even conscious of it. Yet her eyes gave the lie to all that. For there was something behind them concealed by the dull black of their color and yet somehow showing through them; a tenseness, an avid living, such as animals have; which made the woman a complete enigma.

She fascinated me so much that one day as we were working along together at something or other, sweeping I think, an impulse seized me to know this strange woman. It was definite, positive—and I did want to know her. There was something about her I felt a need to understand. In a sudden, impulsive gesture I caught one of her hands and looked full into her face. She returned my gaze; a mysterious expression deepening within her eyes, until I had to avert mine. I cannot describe the look I saw; something so elemental, so age old, so close to the naked soul of things, that the matter-of-fact vocabulary I possess has no words, nor combination of words to describe the offer, and acceptance, of friendship between two "bugs."

Later, when I became better acquainted with her sister I learned something of the life of the two women. At one time there were two sisters and two brothers locked away in this institution. That's a rather high percentage of dements for one pair of parents to turn into the world. Now only the two sisters are left. One of the brothers died in his raving and the other recovered sufficiently to go about his life on the outside. All of them have passed the taint on to others, the Farm-woman is the mother of nine. The sister bore a son sired by her demented brother. She seemed to get some peculiar relief in telling me about it. These were the only times she ever talked in ordinary words.

She said, "One day my brother and I had gone across the creek to haul a truck load of hay. One of my other brothers was driving. When we got loaded and started back around to the bridge, a mile or so away, Joe suggested that we walk back through the creek bottom. Henry was to drive on around and meet us at the barn."

"As soon as we got a little way into the woods, Joe stopped and hugged me. I don't remember if this was the first time or not but things came so easy I guess it must not have been."

"As I said: he hugged me and kissed me, not like a brother, and I liked it; not like a sister, either. His kisses got more and more insistent and he began to fondle me all over."

"It didn't seem to us we were doing anything wrong, we sat down on a pile of leaves and kept right on. I was only about sixteen but all of a sudden I seemed to grow up."

"Henry came back to hunt us. He saw what we were doing and it made him awful mad—'cause we hadn't helped him unload the hay!"

"After that we were together an awful lot, until the folks found out I was pregnant."

"What did you do then?" I asked, and she showed me her back, crisscrossed with scars where her father had beaten her.

"Dad beat me 'til I was almost dead. Then got a doctor to come out to the farm and tend to me."

"When it was born the doctor wasn't going to let me look. He wouldn't let anybody around except another young doctor he brought with him."

"I did look, though. Then I heard somebody screaming. Seemed like I could hear it for days. I can hear it now sometimes. I'm afraid if it doesn't stop, some day it's going to drive me crazy."

"Tell me—what am I doing here? How did I get here? What's become of my father and mother and my brothers? I want them. I don't want any babies. What I saw wasn't a baby anyhow. Make 'em take me home. These people and that howling is driving me crazy. Make 'em take me home."

The whole thing is unthinkable—but they are not responsible for their acts; they are insane. If the sane members of the human race are not interested enough to think for them and take some thought for their children, and their children's children, then have the courage to say who shall be parents, it is not likely the demented members will exercise much wisdom or forethought other than to follow whatever elemental urge they feel at the moment.

One day when Bones was quieter than usual, she stopped before me in her endless stalking and stood eyeing me for a while. I had no idea what was in her mind and I did not speak to her. I had learned that anything she would say was distorted and fantastic. Presently, as though she were as certain of welcome as a favorite child, she crawled into my lap. She seemed so small, helpless and was so confiding in the gesture of seeking comfort in my mothering that my heart swelled with a great ache toward her. I put my arms about her to hold her close. I did not want to fail her and deny her comfort. One of her bone-like arms went about my neck as she laid her head with its brain full of horrors upon my shoulder. I rocked her as I might have rocked a child and for several minutes we sat thus. A response, sympathy and understanding enveloped us and closed down upon us until I do not remember ever sharing a more tender feeling of fellowship with any creature; and it was certainly not founded on any understanding built of words.

I thought of what her life is like now and wondered what it had been like before. As I rocked her, I said to myself, "Poor little girl, I wonder if anyone loved you 'once upon a time.'" No word had been spoken. I had just looked in her face and wondered.

She straightened and I saw a miracle. From somewhere beneath the ever deepening layers of dementia, a memory stole upward clear and plain, bringing with it a beauty that settled in her face, transfiguring it. I looked at her and felt like a trespasser on holy ground. The memory of the thing that had been so lovely, smote the shackles of her Madness from her, and for one breath-taking moment there was an effulgent radiance upon her which transformed her into another person. Even the wildly distorted features were rearranged into another pattern. I was amazed to find she was—beautiful! Her lips moved gently and I had to bend my head to catch the words coming so softly through that rapt, transfigured look.

"Yes, yes—," she spoke with infinite tenderness. "Yes—there was Ralph."

But speaking broke the spell and she slid out of my lap and was gone again—off into some fantastic despair; her fears and phobias are legion—and that is the only time I ever heard her make a rational statement about herself. But I know, for one brief moment, I was allowed to look on something very beautiful.

Now she is lying there asleep in the stupor produced by a drug and the heavy, drawn, unconsciousness of unnatural sleep brings no beauty to her features.

The Farm-woman has gone off the deep end again and is tied down in the side room. I again have her job at the serving table, and have the Pagan and her voracious appetite to contend with. Today at noon she sneaked up behind me, snatched the syrup pitcher and dashed back to her bed with it turned up-side-down above her plate. It overflowed the shallow rim, so as she ran she streamed a broad ribbon of syrup the whole length of the hydro. She has been singing and howling and charging all day. She is raising the roof this minute.

Whew! Just as I finished the sentence about her the nurse came to the door, closed it and told me to put her into a jacket. I did, but I'm puffing like a steam engine. That girl is a wild-cat! The nurse came back just as I was tying the last strap. She seemed surprised I was able to manage her by myself; usually it takes three of us to get her into a jacket. She said the most she expected was that I might be able to divert her attention long enough for her to finish a 'phone call. She asked me if I had suffered any casualties. I hadn't, except I think the Pagan is still grasping a hunk of flesh she pinched out of me, but I don't suppose it's really gone, it just feels like it.

I told her I was afraid I had hurt the girl's arm but she did not go to see about it. If we get hurt in a case like that it is just our hard luck.

Today the Schizo was in one of her moods, sitting at a window she looked up and out with a faraway expression on her otherwise normal face.

I dragged the end of a bed around and sat facing her. Gently I opened a conversation about nothing in particular, then after we had gossiped awhile I asked her:

"You remember you told me you were a 'Juke,' whatever that is, and that you had two strikes on you. Tell me about it, will you?"

She sighed resignedly and answered, "I might as well tell you. I've got to talk to somebody. It may as well be you as one of these others. It's no use trying to talk to the nurses or doctors." She paused, gazing abstractedly into space as I waited.

"Go ahead, tell me, I'm really curious." Then added, to ease her mind, that I might not be as crazy as she thought and later tell about it, "So is Shakespeare."

That did it, turning back to face me, she said:

"Okay, you are going to be here the rest of your 'natural born,' looks like, so you won't be spreading it around outside."

"I'm afraid you are right," I said as she continued.

"'Juke' is the name of a family which has always been a scab on the face of civilization."

"In what way?" I asked.

/167/

She answered moodily, "To begin with that is not their real name. The real name is the same as mine. You know what that is, don't you?"

"Sure, I know what is on your chart. I saw it one day but that means nothing to me," I told her.

"It meant nothing to me either until a few years ago." Again she stopped and gazed out the window, then abruptly turned back and said:

"All my life I've been torn between two entirely different personalities. At least I'll have to call them that for lack of a better word. Whatever it was: I always wanted to do different things."

"Different things?" I said. "That doesn't make you a lunatic."

"Yeah," she answered, "that's just what I expected you to say. I mean I wanted to do different things at the same time."

"Perfectly normal," said I. (There I go, analyzing again). "Everyone has moments of indecision and vacillation."

"Rats," exclaimed 'Schizo' vehemently. "How can I make you understand. You're crazy, too. I couldn't even make the 'psycho' see what I meant. Don't feel bad about it. If he couldn't get it, how could that 'petrified personality' of yours grasp what I mean."

Slightly miffed, I was about ready to drop the subject when she calmed down a little and continued.

"Yes, I told you I had two strikes on me. We'll take 'em in the order of their importance, although in my case the first is now the last; or is that too much like one of your own quotations?"

"Anyway, the 'Jukes' were a family whose history is known back to 1775. That was a name given the descendants of six sisters. They were the daughters of an illiterate Dutch farmer.

One of them had six kids, five of them illegitimate, three of the five were mulatto."

"What's that got to do with you?" I questioned.

"Will you keep still or don't you want me to go ahead. I've decided to get it off my chest to you. It won't cost me anything. You're not goin' anywhere."

"Continue m'Lady," I mumbled meekly. "I'll be quiet. I'm still curious."

"Okay," she said after glancing at me quizzically to see if I was really being sarcastic. "Okay, another sister also had six and four of them were bastards. However, she was a little more careful than Margaret, only two of hers were mulattos. Well to make a long story short, all six of them were about alike. Most of their male offspring were feeble minded and all of the females of that generation became prostitutes."

"All?" I queried.

"All," she said, "yes, all."

"The same thing has been going on ever since. Along about 1875 some professor was made Commissioner of Charities and Corrections or some such title. He noticed a great similarity in names of inmates in the jails, poor-houses and penitentiaries. It only took him a little while to get deeply into this."

"He found, at that time, more than fifteen hundred descendants of the six girls. I can give you percentages and statistics till the moon comes over the mountain. For instance, seventy-three per cent of all these people were illegitimate. Ten of them were murdered. Three-fourths of the women were whores, seven-tenths of the men were petty crooks, drunkards or paupers. Only once in a great while was one of them of average intelligence. Seven hundred and ninety-six persons had married into the

'Jukes.' Their offspring, too succumbed to the syphilitic taint of the family."

"I know the family, you see. I studied it in school but after I found out I was one of them I really got down to business and boned up on my ancestors. If any of them were on the Mayflower it should have been sunk before it landed."

"Yes, but how do you know you are a 'Juke'? You said that was the name given them by this professor."

"I'm coming to that," she said. "Gimme time. Wait'll I tell you about the rapists; about the mothers who operated 'houses' with their daughters as inmates. About the incest they committed, sometimes with mere children. And don't let me forget to tell you about the fathers who pimped for their daughters. When they weren't using them themselves, I mean."

"And the blindness, yeah the blind were numerous in our family. An average, according to this professor, Dugdale was his name, of a hundred and twenty-three per thousand. Ordinary people have about three to a thousand."

"But you said that beautiful body of yours was your inheritance. It doesn't sound to me like a family with mulatto blood, with syphilis and blindness and interbreeding would produce very much beauty," I said. "I should think they would be everything else but pretty."

"That's just one of those things," she replied. "Most of the women were, if not beauties, at least goodlooking and nearly all of them had curves just like mine. Maybe that accounts for them being such successful prostitutes."

"It's an odd thing," she went on, "but while the females are above average in looks they mostly had no brains. Just bodies. The men were not goodlooking, most of them were morons and showed it. As far as the interbreeding's concerned, the original clan, back there in those rock hills, did interbreed and even intermarried."

"It seemed that the girls never married until they had two or three little bastards. Then they'd marry and have some more kids. Some of the family did drift away from the old "stamping grounds" though, and married outsiders. A few of these became ordinary people. This guy Dugdale had chased down seven generations, (just to see if that other quotation of yours was right, I guess) and found 'em all alike, except those few I mentioned."

"Occasionally a bunch of kids would be taken away from their parents and adopted out. Some of these turned out alright and some of 'em just followed the ways of their forefathers. There was one of 'em called Eve, after one of the original six sisters, not the woman who wore the fig leaf, this one wasn't so bashful. She had four or five kids, some of 'em by escaped slaves, some of 'em by so-called 'Gentlemen' and some of 'em by her foster brothers, cousins or whoever was handy when she took a notion. She had been sent to a 'boarding' family in another county but notice how she followed the pattern."

"How do you know you are one of them?" I asked. "Surely their name was concealed."

"Sure it was concealed," she replied. "I just happen to be one of the few whose name has remained the same through a crooked, weaving line of descension. That is, I'm a daughter of the males."

"Well, that doesn't explain how you found out the name, does it?" I questioned.

"I told you there was one who became famous, didn't I?"

"Yes," I said, "you did. What does that prove?"

"His name was the same as mine. He wrote a play. That's what made him famous. This play was about the rest of the family. He even sent about a hundred tickets to his relatives," she answered.

"When he was about sixty he broke his arm. It wouldn't heal; on account of his syphilitic blood, I guess, so he killed himself," she continued. "There was quite a story about it in some old newspapers I found. With these bits of information and my own inclinations, which were driving me to distraction, I checked into it and found out I was a 'Juke.' Then I knew what made me like I am."

"That's a lot of hooey," I said, "you just let your imagination run away with you."

"Imagination. That's what you think," she stated viciously. "I know what I'm talking about. My father and mother had left the old neighborhood miles behind. We had moved out here and lived in a small town. We were poor as church mice, but father never would do much about it. Just said, 'It will all come out all right.' Most of my brothers and sisters were slow in school. I wasn't. I wanted an education so I could get out and go places."

"You sound like you got it," I said in a flattering manner.

"Sure, I got it," she answered. "Got through high school. Then the war came on and I went to France with the Red Cross. I was proud of myself then; proud to be a part of the A.E.F. under Pershing. At that time, you see, I didn't know about the 'Jukes.' It was the other 'strike' which bothered me in those days. That's why I said the first shall be last. Together they were too much for me."

The Schizo began to get a wild look in her eyes. She arose and started pacing back and forth. I decided to let her alone for a few minutes, hoping she would continue. She didn't; just kept on getting worse and worse. She began talking to herself and tearing at her forehead with her hands.

Soon the nurse came, saw her and phoned for a jacket. The Schizo was tied down.

The Pagan is such a beautiful girl it is heart-breaking to see her so! She has been here a long time. Before I was sent to the hydro I often heard the patients up on the ward discussing her. They were filled with hot resentment at what they thought this place had done to her. She was apparently completely recovered and was expecting to be released to go home. All summer and fall she waited, poised and controlled—and had so much charm she was a general favorite with the others, and very popular. So much so that there were none who spoke of her without showing the bitterness and resentment they felt toward whatever their varying ideas of "fate" were. To quote one of them specifically:

"If you want an example of what this place will do to a person go down there to the hydro and see that girl! Prettiest thing that ever walked on two feet, and absolutely the sweetest girl I ever knew in my life! And what happened to her? She was up here for months and months; perfectly straight and well; and how did they treat her? Every day they told her that she could 'go home soon.' Every day she waited and waited."

"I do not know what the trouble was, whether her people did not want her, or whether the doctors would not let her go. They just kept putting her off like they do everybody, telling you nothing you can depend on for the truth! Why, she thought she was going to get to go home for the Fourth of July! Then she thought sure she would get to go home for her birthday. Then for Thanksgiving! Thankgiving came and she had her dinner here with the rest of us."

"Then when Christmas came; she had been so sure she would be with her people for that! She got along well enough till the middle of the afternoon on Christmas day—and she just got so homesick she couldn't stand it any longer. She cracked. So they took her down to the hydro. But the sanest person who ever lived would go nuts in this place!"

"I'd like to see some of these doctors and nurses who think they have such damned fine minds locked up and treated as we are. If they could pass an intelligence test when they were called to that 'clinic,' I'd take my hat off to them and admit they are as smart as they think they are! No wonder we don't act like human beings! They don't treat us like human beings—and after a while we get the same ideas ourselves!"

That speech came from one of those up on the "best" ward. I do not know how straight her reasoning was; for she too, had been adjudged insane.

But we do have to adjust ourselves somehow to the strange system we are ruled by. The easiest way is to admit you are a nut —and go ahead and live down to it. They who are entirely insane fare better than those who are only half-cracked. There are no premiums on intelligence in this place. And for personal comfort and possible hope of recovery I prefer it down here with the maniacs, rather than trying to live up on the "best" ward. Its advantages are highly over-rated. And never again will I make the effort I made at one time to be a "model" patient.

A nurse was dismissed on the spot when a doctor happened to see her slap a patient. His seeing it was an accident. There would not be many left on the staff if all of them just happened to be caught at some of their practices. With my own eyes I have seen worse things than just slapping a patient.

One of the nurses told me she would see to it that I was not reported if I would "pick a quarrel" with a patient whom she particularly disliked and "beat her to death." She thought I was insane enough to do it, but I was not—even if I was at that time trying very hard to be a "model" patient; and doing as all the other patients do who have a spark of sanity. They range themselves as satellites around the star of their choice and do all in their power to uphold the ludicrous feudal system which is a vest-pocket edition of some ancient barony. A feudal system set up under the very laws of the state, which thrives and flourishes here in the middle of modern America.

Endless conniving—not to say downright lying; petty intrigues; treachery, on a lilliputian scale. Gossip—so small the narrowest Main street in the smallest town in the country would not stoop to repeat it. If we are model patients we must do all in our power to uphold the traditions. Wash and mend the nurse's clothes on the sly—for that is not supposed to be allowed. Buy their favor with our adulation; and their favor is sold to the one who can apply the smoothest coating of flattery. I have been spoken of as a "good" patient. I abominate myself for the despicable "yes-lady" I had to be to earn their approval.

One patient raised a devil of a ruckus up on one of the other wards when a patient, especially unpopular with the nurse, was put into a jacket and left lying on the floor. That was not so bad—strait-jackets are a universal experience in this odd world; they are accepted more or less as a matter of course. But when they had her tied down they were not through with her. The nurse stood by and let two other patients jump upon her, kicking and trampling her under their feet. The woman who told me the story rushed up and pushed them off. The nurse caught her, shook her and told her that if she did not "mind her own business" she would be put into a jacket herself!

The woman stood her ground and threatened to report it to the doctor, but the nurse did not interfere with the two who were doing the kicking. However the other woman had more courage than most patients. She shook the nurse and told her it would mean her job if the woman was hurt; she meant to talk.

I asked her if she told the doctor and she looked at me pityingly. "Don't you know how much our word is not worth?"

But she did bluff the nurse, and she called her dogs off. It did not get to the doctor; patients don't tell. There were none of the woman's bones broken—she was only bruised and they were not in places which showed.

One nurse was dismissed for slapping a patient—but with my own eyes I saw another strike a patient in the pit of the stomach with her fist.

A little girl mother, not yet out of her teens, was sent here almost before she was able to be up after her confinement. She lay in bed in a condition of abject terror so shrinking and pitiful it made the heart stop to see her. I do not know what the thing was she feared so; but it gripped her till she could not speak and her eyes were too tragic to look at. The nurse ordered her brought to the bathroom to have her breasts cared for (she had been nursing her baby and they were heavy and painful). However, she was conscious of no pain except the terror gripping her.

Two of the other patients and I went in to get her. She shrank away and cowered as though we had come to lead her to torture. She did not try to fight us, just whimpered and shuddered and cowered so we had to drag her from the bed by force. As we dragged her along, her fingers caught at everything they touched and clung till the bones were nearly broken. A fourth patient stepped up and removed her gripping fingers from the door frame as we went through. Then went along with us rather than tear the fingers from their clinging grip on her own hand.

When we got her into the bathroom, the nurse was impatient

because we had been so long in bringing her, as none of us had the heart to be brusque and unkind with her. She told her to sit down, but the girl had no comprehension left to understand anything; her fear had filled every part of her brain and consumed it. We all saw she did not comprehend; so one of the others put her hands on her shoulders, and I stooped down to bend her knees to seat her. She had clasped her hands tightly before her face in a gesture of pleading but her eyes were so filled with terror she did not even see us, and her body was rigid with it.

"Let her alone! I told her to sit down and she is going to without any help from anybody! Sit down!" The voice was harsh but anyone could see the command had not registered.

One of the others again placed her hands on the girl's shoulders. The nurse was furious. She turned to the other—and her face was not good to look at.

"Did you hear what I said? Let her alone! I guess I'm still running this ward and I'll put you in a jacket if you don't learn to mind me!" Then to the other:

"Sit Down! I said: Sit Down! Are you going to or not!" But the girl had no comprehension.

"All right, I guess you want me to make you! Well, you asked for it. Here, take it!" She took deliberate aim and hit the young mother full in the pit of the stomach! The girl dropped with a grunt as the breath was expelled from her. Otherwise she did not change her expression as there was nothing left in her not consumed in the throes of her terror. She did not know she had been the victim of the petty, vindictive rage of another.

The nurse stood over her tugging at her breasts like a farmhand milking a cow and the milk streamed into a washpan. I never saw a breast-pump in the whole institution; for all I know

/177/

this may be the best method—but not the way it's done here. If breasts must be cared for it is done in a very barbarous fashion. She accompanied the milking with a vindictive tirade lost altogether on the other.

Occasionally injustices happen in one of these institutions which arouse the public ire—but nothing can check countless little underhanded, nagging, dirty things done. I am certain those in charge of us do the very best they can with the material they have to work with. The hours of work are long and hard—the pay is poor and people who can do better do not choose to be nut-herds in an insane asylum. Most of them are very ignorant. Few even have a high school education. One of them had two years of training in a small hospital and that gives her a very high rating of superiority over the others. It also increases the size of her pay envelope. She is paid the astounding sum thirty-five dollars a month for a six-day week, twelve hours a day. The others are paid thirty dollars a month.

I do not know whether asylum work only attracts people of a certain mental make-up; or whether the work develops it in them—but to save me, I can see nothing in most of them to warrant the exalted idea they have of their own unquestionable superiority. Many of them had risen no higher than domestic help when they too were on the "outside." One came from a laundry, another was a waitress. Those are honest occupations, and essential, not to be ashamed of; but I cannot see (I admit I am insane, but I still cannot see) why they are such superior people!

But here where there are none but the inferior for comparison, they shine in their own eyes very brightly; so they stay.

The things they do which reveal their petty tyranny and cruelty are not great acts of wrong-doing needing public redression. They are acts of petty vindictiveness; revealing how shriveled and small the human soul can become if exposed to the dehydrating experience of dealing with dements. The treachery, conniving, and lying going on among them for the notice and approbation of those in authority is pitiful.

There is a new patient who is painfully conscious of embarrassment when exposed. She is in a strait-jacket with no garments under it. The nurse just now brought her a bed pan and ripped back the sheet covering her. The woman protested at being exposed. The answer the nurse made her was as crude as some of the language the patients use. Such modesty is only a senseless phobia as far as the nurse is concerned—and because of it she will do what she can to make the other suffer. Modesty is a mighty poor asset here and the sooner it is dispensed with, the better. The hydro is the nakedest place in the world but it does seem the nurse might have spread the sheet back over the woman!

But she didn't. She took it to use about one of the other patients and the woman is still lying there naked. I cannot prevent the resentment from rising within me.

Perhaps it is just a senseless phobia but I'm damned if I don't cover her up if the nurse does not bring the sheet back in just a half-minute! Then got myself rudely cut down upon for interfering.

The nurse is coming back with a fresh sheet but is not going to spread it over the woman just yet! Something or other attracted her attention outside and she went to the window. She has the sheet in her hand but has walked the length of the dormitory to look out another window. She is serenely unconscious of the woman's flaming face; exaggeratedly unconscious. Going out of her way to make it pointed! And this sheet of paper is about to be crumpled up in my hand for I can do nothing about it. But I'm damned if I can hold myself down much longer.

I want to rip every garment off her! If I interfere I will be reported as "disturbed" for the nurse is sane; I am insane; and "Three Building" is yawning wide for me. I guess I had better go ask for a jacket. The woman is crying, but what does that matter. She is, after all, only a nut.

I can say truthfully I have never been the least bit mistreated but I cannot say so much about some of the others who did not have the good fortune to be constructed along the architectural lines of an Amazon. In ancient days when the whole world was in a state of barbarism and savagery, a powerful physique was a most valuable asset. Here in a bug-house, where all civilization has slipped back into the Dark Ages pattern, it has that same value.

Why do they not treat us all alike and let us all feel the lash of their authority in the same manner? Why do they not yank and yell at me and the Medicine-maker as they do the others? We have each failed to pass a sanity test. Why do they not approach us in the same insulting manner as they do some of the others? Why do they shake us and twist our arms—and break them? One woman had her arm broken down here. If keeping the patients cowed with fear; if charging about, threatening them and carrying the threats out as far as the laws of the state will tolerate, resorting to countless petty insults and dirty underhanded things, is the best way to manage those who are demented, then why are we three, the Medicine-maker, the Farm-woman and I, excepted?

The woman whose arm was broken is an example of the type they choose. One night, the nurse (who did not know how to change a bed)—was putting the patients to bed with the customary yanking, yelling and pushing. The bluff system had worked so well with the woman she feared that particular nurse more than the Devil. Because she was shrinking and timorous the nurse caught her, flung her into bed and told her to stay there.

The woman had not been raving, nor was she violently disturbed at the time. The nurse just treated her so because it pleased her sense of power. As the night wore away the patient lay sleepless and staring; not taking her eyes off the nurse. Finally she asked her why she didn't go to sleep. The woman answered that her arm was hurting and she could not sleep. The nurse railed out that she would "hurt more than her arm if she did not turn over and go to sleep." Sleep did not come for the woman, but the nurse paid her no further notice. Next morning when the day nurse came on duty they noticed something wrong with the woman's arm; it bulged and hung helpless. When the doctor came he found it broken.

All this happened before my transfer down here—and the nurse herself told me about it. Told it with relish that she had been able to make her power felt to such an extent over another. It was very like bragging! She said the woman would lie in her bed for hours, not saying a word—"she was afraid to!"

I was curious about the incident and asked the nurse questions. She was in an expansive mood when she told me and I tried to get her viewpoint. Though the woman is in her grave now and I never saw her; still, I can see nothing to it that should give the nurse pleasure.

"The woman looked at me all the time with the funniest look on her face," she said, "sometimes it would give me the creeps. Once I asked her why she kept looking at me and she said, without batting an eye,

"You are the one who broke my arm, and you know it!"

/181/

"I told her, sure I broke your arm—and I'll break the other one if you don't quit your staring!"

"I was really sorry I had done it—still I could not let her know it. I wouldn't have done it but I guess I have more strength than I know. I could not let her know it had been an accident. I wanted her to think I had done it on purpose. She never gave me any more trouble. She had never been a bad patient anyway —but I did not want her to get the idea that it mattered."

And then they wonder why we do not act like "human beings."

There is no way such a condition can be changed. We have let our civilization slip. We must be governed by the only system the world was able to devise when it was all in the same condition.

We, who are insane, are people whom the rest of the world has washed its hands of. We are the untouchables and must be controlled by those who are willing to pay the price for their work—and they do pay a huge price for it.

They come among us and do the best they can with a people whom the rest of the world could not stand to look at—or touch with a forty foot pole. If Utopia ever does come I do not suppose it will be set up in the world as an insane asylum. And the people who care for us are—only people.

I am going to try to remember that, and not let my resentment at the petty little things get my viewpoint all out of focus. It is so easy to slip on a pair of indigo spectacles! And when they are worn the whole world is very, very blue indeed. But I do wish they would deal a little more frankly with us. Even when we try to cooperate with them—they put obstacles hard to climb over in our way and very often there is glaring evidence that they resent and discourage any presumption that we are still human beings.

The trouble they have with the patients is fostered as much by the false attitude they have toward us, as it is by our insanity. For it is imperative that they deal frankly with those not too well supplied with reasoning faculties. Why they should go about building distorted ideas in the minds of the patients is beyond my comprehension. They try to make us think they have unlimited power over us without any check. That is not true, or there would not be a supervisor or a doctor who makes two trips a day through the wards.

And though there may be a slip and a patient's arm may be broken, still I have the feeling that we are safe from any great harm. The very fact of their jealousy and intrigue makes for our safety as nothing so very bad could be done without them reporting it among themselves. It is everybody for himself in this strange system—and the devil take the hindmost!

The night nurses, even here in the hydro where the wildly demented are sent, cannot put one of us in a strait-jacket without an order from the supervisor. Nor can they give us so much as a dose of salts without a doctor's order. So in reality, the power they have over us is a myth. Perhaps that is why they struggle so hard to create the illusion of it. Because it is only an illusion when you come right down to the facts in the case, and they know it. They do not like to have it known to us they are powerless. But as long as control of this institution is in the hands of the present officials, I shall not fear greatly to be sent even to the bleak imprisonment of "Three Building." I have seen enough of the doctors—and especially the day supervisor to know they are human beings; not ogres—not monsters.

I saw the doctor's eyes when he looked down on the little sick girl—and they were the eyes of a feeling fellow creature. And the very day that I came to this institution, the day supervisor stood over me, put her hand on my knee and looked full into my face, and I saw the frank gaze of a kind and wise woman. If the time ever comes that I must go to "Three Building," I shall go without fear, remembering her. For I have seen her eyes—and I have seen the way these others step to live up to the things she demands of them. As long as I know she is somewhere in the institution and will look in on the condition of our surroundings twice daily, I will go where I am sent with no very great fear for the outcome. She has enough integrity for the whole bunch. She does much to fill in the lack of some of the others, and so give the entire staff a fairly high average.

Some of those whose authority exceeds that of the nurses are not completely untouched by the taint of small, narrow practices. One trifling example came when a new patient was being admitted. She was still in the office while the papers that consigned her here were being signed. The doctor who received her is probably a high standing member of his profession. I do not know. But when the woman asked him casually if she would be allowed to smoke when the door closed upon her, she was answered very positively in the affirmative,

"Sure! You can have all the cigarettes you want!"—when he knew very positively that smoking is forbidden the women. The men are allowed to smoke—and if they have no money with which to buy tobacco, it is furnished them by the state. But the women—that is another matter! Even if they have their own money with which to buy their cigarettes, they cannot have them—it is "immoral" for women to smoke. But they may have snuff! And if they have no money with which to buy it—they will be supplied it out of state funds. So they who want cigarettes must learn to dip snuff instead—for it is immoral to smoke. If they become too nervous because of the sudden denial—they will be given drugs! But no matter—that is just one of the odd customs in this medieval arrangement.

CHAPTER *12*

THE WOMAN WITH the unbelievably high temperature is being transferred to the hospital. All the time she has been down here she has rolled her head and talked about "seeing her mistake." Nothing is known about her except that she, her husband and a tiny new-born baby were traveling west when she became sick and demented. How she could have such a high temperature and not be at least delirious, whether insane or not, I do not know. Nor do I understand why anyone as sick as she evidently is, should be sent to a hospital for the insane. With a temperature like that it would seem she belonged in a hospital where the nurses at least know how to change beds! I know nothing of medicine but believe she is a victim of the ancient plague which attended child-birth before modern medicine discovered a way to lessen the high mortality at delivery. I have helped care for her and saw enough to indicate that something is terribly wrong with her—and it is not in her head!

It seems like a colossal mistake on somebody's part! Some sanity commission passed on her before sending her here. I wonder if there were no thermometers among the doctors who examined her? To send a woman with a terrible temperature to the hydro, into all this racket and uproar, because she was talking out of her head with a temperature of one hundred and ten degrees is criminal and to be cared for by "nurses" who only have the experience of teachers, laundry workers and waitresses is even worse. They may not have time to get around to her before the infection has killed her—and if she does live long enough for them to examine her—they will test her mentality. Unless her blood-test shows a positive "Wassermann" the matter will be ended. Perhaps they will do more for her at the hospital but she has been down here about forty-eight hours, in a strait-jacket; and every minute is precious in fighting the infection. Down here are "nurses" who know nothing of nursing—only of strait-jackets. As helpers they have only such nuts as are loose at the time. Even the supervisors have risen to the position since they started the care of the demented. I do not believe there is a registered nurse on the whole staff, with the possible exception of the one in charge of the hospital. As helpers she has some of the better patients!

And while I believe those who are here are doing the best they can to care for the people under them, sometimes things happen that might be a small matter to people who lived where they were not quite so helpless. If a doctor happens to make a mistake—and all people make mistakes—even such superior creatures as doctors in insane asylums, there is no appeal and no escape from it. It is just the patient's hard luck—we have no say in any matter and the breath we expend in trying to express an opinion might as well be used for something else. Nothing we say is of any consequence.

Upon the "best" ward is a girl who told me her story. She lay for nearly a week in a strait-jacket. She admitted she belonged there since she was literally mad with pain in her side. But the doctor dismissed it as "hysteria"—said she was only "disturbed" and left her lying there day after day. He was so sure of his diagnosis he did not even take the trouble to look at her side.

She stood in better with the superintendent—and when he came through on his Sunday inspection she asked him to examine her. He took one look, rushed to the phone and ordered the hospital staff to prepare immediately for an emergency operation. There was not a moment to lose. The girl was in a critical condition from acute appendicitis!

I do not know whether her story is true. The girl has been adjudged insane. But I do know and I have been pronounced insane too, of another woman up on the "best" ward whose blood test showed an amazing syphilitic content. Of course, she is being given "shots." However, nothing was done when she complained of acute local discomfort until one of the other patients raised a complaint about the revolting odor clinging to her. The nurse fixed up a douche and called another patient to administer it to her. It was given in the stool-room, publicly and very carelessly and the operation was accompanied with lewdness and ribald remarks which may have been very amusing to those who care for that type of entertainment. Thereafter the woman was given a douche every few days; the time for them being determined by the olfactory offense to the others. One patient consoled her most practically:

"Don't worry," she said, "they will do something for you when you get so rotten and stinking nobody can stand you!"

The night nurses are on duty again and are pulling the beds of the noisiest patients out into the day-hall trying to separate the sheep from the goats—those who are raving from those not making quite so much noise in the hope the almost quiet ones will go to sleep. Personally, I would prefer the noise of their raving to the atrocious racket the metal bedposts make as they are dragged across the cement; especially the Camel's bed; when the Camel is on it. It is a little low bed of solid iron and takes three people straining like oxen to budge it. The Camel loves the little low bed and always gets it if she can. She has been in a jacket raving her lungs out and just now as they pulled her past, her strident caliope voice sounded high above the bed-post accompaniment:

"O-o-o-h! O-o-o-o-h! Now what are you doing this for?—Pulling me out here with all these crazy people! Taking me for a crazy buggy ride." (She is not wrong there—for the trip from dormitory to day-hall across this shrieking concrete is a "crazy buggy ride" alright!)

"Shame on you! Shame on you! Putting me out here with these crazy people! Shame on you. I'll show you though; I'll show you. You watch and see if I don't show you! You'll be ashamed of yourselves then. First you put me in a horse jacket and drag me around like a jack-ass in a halter. You won't even dust me with flea powder to kill the fleas. Why don't you lead me out and back me up against this buggy you make me ride in. I'd show you some real paces. Listen at 'em holler! Listen at 'em holler—git along little dogie—I'm a bein' tuk to th' l-a-s-t round-up. In Bill Murray's horse jacket. And they are all blind drunk! Listen to 'em holler!"

"Nurse, nurse, if you want to make some money I'm the nag to bet on! Put your money on me! Put your money on me! They can stay awake and holler all night if they want to, but I am going to sleep, and sleep like a little white lamb. I'll show you; just like a little white lamb!"

She will probably lead in the raving; her lungs are made of leather! Now she is singing, "When Shadows Fall" and her voice is more like a caliope than ever. There is neither melody nor music in her singing. She opens her mouth wide and releases whatever sound happens to come out. Then hangs on to it as long as she can.

It is bed-time for us all. Another day has passed, and every day is just one more day gone. There are no yesterdays that are safe to think about; no tomorrows which can be thought of with any safety either. Only today; this minute; an hour at a time. The memory of other evenings when things were different, does not bring any peace. Neither do the days stretching ahead. They will be no different. Only today. It is all that can be borne. If it is endurable, life must flow on in a shallow and meaningless channel scarcely called living.

And now the morning. Another day to live through. There were no drugs given through the night so now this place is a bedlam. It is usually quieter in the morning—but not this morning. A boiler factory would be as silent as a morgue by comparison. The shrieking bed-posts in transit add their quota of ear-splitting racket to the already insufferable uproar. Even the nurses look a little wild as they go charging about trying to keep the whip lash of their authority, but it has lost its sting—the whole place is stark mad.

Those who are tied down are howling and shrieking—and those who are loose are racing and charging about and adding wild gesticulations to their howls and shrieks. They all seem like bare trees in a forest through which the wind of their madness is sweeping; bowing them, bending them, breaking them. It is the wildest hysteria imaginable. I do not know what happened. But some virulent contagion swept among them—spreading, it is catching me too.

Their madness excites the madness in me to higher and higher pitches—and presently I shall be howling too. I do not have the power to resist the hysteria and bedlam which has broken loose this morning. It is worse than Hell. Dante knew nothing about it. He should have made his memorable trip through a hydro when chaos and destruction were riding! He would have found enough material to fill many volumes.

The beautiful naked Pagan has slipped out of her jacket and is standing at a window, howling at the morning. I am certain Dante heard nothing in Hell more blood-curdling than the howls and shrieks tearing the vocal cords from her throat; shattering the ear drums of all who must hear her. My own brain is quivering on the verge of dissolution. Nothing can retain a definite contour when it is subjected to an explosion such as we have this morning.

I cannot stand it! Shakespeare! For God's sake, where are you! Sit here and help me hang on to this pencil! I tell you I cannot stand it. I feel the roots of my hair drawing together so I know it is standing on end and the flesh of my arms is all goosebumps. Feel of my hair, Mr. Shakespeare, and tell me if it is not standing on end—no never mind, I know it is. But no matter—you just hang on to this pencil and write something; write it fast for we cannot afford to lift our voices even one little peep. You hang on to this pencil and put something on paper. Anything—anything! I am not going to lift my voice in this howling. You do not like nuts, do you, Mr. Shakespeare? They are not nearly so interesting when you are one of them and have to live, see, and hear them when there are no others for variation. I cannot say I like them either, but I know I am as insane as the wildest one here. I cannot afford to let it be known by howling out loud. Sorry, Mr. Shakespeare; you should not have come to me so blithely as my delusion of grandeur. I know it was more pleasant back in your quiet English grave.

You did not know what sort of a jam you were getting yourself into. But now you are here I cannot turn you loose to let you go back; much as I would like to go with you. I cannot stand this and I dare not dismiss you. Your education is being completed, Mr. Shakespeare. Now you can write about nuts from experience—first hand experience and you will not have to depend upon your more comfortable imagination. I know when you build characters from fancy they are more pleasant but here they are all around you charging, howling, and no one—not even you with your former skillful use of language, could construct such creatures with words—for words cannot portray them.

This is the real thing, Mr. Shakespeare. Madness. Stark, senseless, maniacal Madness. It is like a mad bull in a pasture—much safer when you can survey it through a tall fence, from a safe distance. Unless you write faster; you will be tossed on the horns of the creature; to say nothing of being gored and trampled. You are seeing Madness here, Mr. Shakespeare; at first hand—and you have nothing but the stub of a chewed up pencil to protect yourself with. You will sure as hell have to write faster. I'm going—I feel that crazy "light" feeling in the temples and my eyes are not seeing things rightly. Write, damn it. Write something. Anything, it does not matter.

There is something around my head so tight I cannot think, but you are going to sit here and keep putting something on paper. That is the law and I'm laying it down to you. You shall not run out on me. I need you now if I ever needed you. And remember, Mr. Shakespeare, one little squawk and your goose will be cooked. You are not a genius in this present inferno, only a nut in a bug-house. So it need not make the least bit of difference what you write; just so you keep at it. I cannot help you with it—for I feel my brain exploding. For God's sake keep at it! Never mind whether it is something you would like to say—or whether it has any beauty. You have no time to use an eraser if you had one.

Keep writing—and write as though you were pursued by Satan —for whether you have sense enough to know it or not—you are! Something has caught us and is sweeping us to the devil. You are not writing drama this time, you are living it.

Get busy, "Three Building" is worse than this. You are not preserving the best traditions of English literature now—it is a few glimmers and shreds of reason you hold together—if you can. It is your sanity you are trying to rescue.

Write faster—you fool—if you do not want to disintegrate into a jittering idiot. Your reason has left you already and the only thing keeping you from becoming another howling maniac is just not turning loose and being one; for you certainly have the makings of a real one. Keep on with your writing. Do not run out on me—I know I cannot make the grade without you.

If you can keep me from howling it will be a greater indication of genius than anything possibly conjured out of the imagination. This is not imagination—it is worse. It is a nightmare. A nightmare while you are wide awake, so no one can come awaken you if you yell. Wide awake in the middle of a nightmare, Mr. Shakespeare. If you were asleep you might yell and maybe someone would hear you, come in and shake you—but if you yell in this—all the shaking they can give you will not awaken you. Mr. Shakespeare—My God! Do you want to yell? Well—don't! Shut it up before it gets started, damn it.

I told you to write—write you fool! Words! Anything! Never mind whether or not they make sense. Write! Shut up and say it on paper! You are a bigger jack-ass than I. Genius—Bah! Nut —brother nut! Whatever genius you may have had you lost coming to me. You damned fool, if you give way to this hysteria and let so much as one little peep out of you there will be no stopping it. I know—I had that happen once, and no power on earth can stop it. The only way to hold it is to stop it before it gets started. The primeval chaos had nothing on this—it was as sedate as a middle-aged spinster. Poor Bill, poor Bill; what a jamb for a genius to get into.

Come next time to someone who wants to write about the flowers, birds and bees, William, for there is nothing this side of Hell like Madness. But hold the fort for a few minutes longer. The rescue is coming! The rescue is coming: in the form of a nurse, God bless her, and Mercury, dear God of speed, help her to hurry! She has a hypodermic in each hand and another nurse is bringing a cup of paraldehyde. God bless and prosper the man who discovered it! Drugs—Drugs—Unconsciousness! Quietness!

Well—that was that, William. We made it! Thank you! I have no idea what you have written the last few minutes—but I know I feel like Jacob of old who contended with the angel. I have an ankle out of joint and am so wringing wet with perspiration there is not a dry thread upon me. I am most grateful to you. The doctor can give my sick hypo to someone who did not have the good fortune to choose you for a delusion of grandeur. He can think what he likes of delusions of grandeur—but what you did for me, I could not do for myself. We made it! Whether the world ever knows it or not—the writing you have been doing for the last half hour is an indication of greater genius than all your previous works put together!

Shakespeare, we got through that crisis—though it seemed for awhile it would happen and in spite of everything I was going to go off at the deep end—with a splash. When and if that happens there is only "Three Building" left—and hopeless insanity.

Since you have filled many pages with so much that is somber —are there no lighter hues to look upon? I am tired of such gloom—is there no lightness and laughter? Surely all the world is not filled with tragedy; or is it? Is there nothing in this world but maniacs raving in madness? Shakespeare, I tell you I cannot stand it! It is better to throw up my hands and sink into "Three Building." The way it seems now it does not make much difference which way the fall is—just to get off the fence one way or the other! I am tired of straddling endless fences. If I must be a maniac—why not be a real one? What is the advantage of this half-measure?

Madness itself has a few compensations. With all of my trying where do I get? Just putting off for a little while longer that which is inevitable—I cannot avert it. It will come. It will claim me sometime—sooner or later. So what's the use in trying to defer it? It's a senseless effort to try and escape the inescapable.

Bah! Shakespeare—what a bust you are turning out to be. That sort of thinking never helped anyone. If you can do no better than that you might just as well end your writing. I can do more than enough of that sort of thinking. Find me something cheerful to think of; something pleasant to look at. I have seen so much of madness and horror and chaos my own eyes are streaming with it so it settles upon everything I look at. I see nothing but the horror filling my own eyes. Nothing can reach into my brain around it; it obstructs all other seeing. I would rather tear my brain from my skull with my own hands than see any more of it.

I can understand now how the girl felt who was locked in the side-room, alone with her madness; in such despair that she tried vainly to rip her skull apart. In three days she had torn every strand of hair out by the roots, handful by handful. This left her head as bald as her palm; and still she tore at it in the starkest madness imaginable.

But, Shakespeare, she recovered! She did! And her triumph has encouraged many. She did not wind up on "Three Building." Even now she is going about her life on the "outside" still minus her hair. Never was there another quite so insane as she. Yet she recovered! All things have an end sometime or other; nothing goes on unchanged forever. Anything can be endured for awhile, even Madness—and life in the hydro. At that it is better and easier to live down here with the maniacs than on the "best" ward, which is the most highly overrated place imaginable!

Upstairs on the "best" ward sit those who have only a mild form of madness. They live, they move, they have their being in a congested furore of suppression. Their days come and go, making scarcely enough ripple on the surface of time to mark their passing. Existence is geared to a monotony grinding on and on interminably.

Each day is like its predecessor—and all the tomorrows will be no different. Each day is filled with the same bustle and importance of preparing for the doctor's and supervisor's rounds. All that is needed to complete the illusion of military precision is to hear "company! 'ten-shun!'"

Back of the preparation and bustle; behind the institutional orderliness; behind the precision of forty chairs evenly spaced and forty beds arranged in perfect geometric parallel; behind the perfection of well modulated human voices (whose owners must see to it they stay perfectly modulated—that being the price of staying on the best ward—and damn the best ward)—back of all the numerous perfections of the best ward, there is a stalking, mawkish, nightmarish knowledge that the whole thing is insane, senseless and stupid—and oh, so hopeless. But that knowledge is carefully hidden from the ones who live there.

Of course there are those who do see it—and in their seeing lose the right to stay there. They are at once transferred to some other ward to be with those who also have seen hope depart. Their transfer does not matter to them nor does anything have any meaning; they are then quite mad. Life, freedom, kindred, family and friends; all things which mean "living" to humanity lose all importance and cease to be for the patient deserted by hope.

When Madness comes—a strange anaesthesia follows. A sleep akin to death, but more mysterious. A rest from the dim regions of unconsciousness—a state which is neither death nor living; lethal, mysterious—evil perhaps to some, but only to those who do not know the blind, intolerable horror that comes from seeing something which cannot be borne—nor escaped.

What matter if this thing bringing stark madness to one frail creature might perchance be a problem another mind could take in easy stride? Before the lesser consciousness gave way to shrieks and tearing hair; to curses violent to hear; or laughter, the soul the small mind dwelt in knew to its full and complete capacity all the night-marish terror it was capable of feeling. Until emotion rising, like water in a trap, tripped a release somewhere along its many devious channels, and gushed out in the turbulent, unchecked and uncheckable flow called Madness.

Sometimes the break comes slowly. A pressure unmarked at the first, but slowly rising. A gnawing discontent; a childish fear that swings onward and outward in an ever widening orbit etching itself into the mysterious force called personality. Perhaps it is such a small, slow motion when it first begins that the beginning is lost sight of. Then Ruin follows. For Ruin it most surely is; as any know who have stood beside a fellow being strapped hand and foot to save himself and others from his fury. We call it Ruin; this collapse of faculties where reason is displaced by demoniac delusions; where staid and ordered thought gives way and in the "ordered track of reason, a wild disorder reigns and all the senses riot." Ruin.

However, like all other happenings, the viewpoint modifies the scene. I who stand on the other side of this phenomenon called Madness, would like to stretch a hand across to those who may some day, go through it. Or (may God spare them!) stand by someone they love and watch the barrier rising; see the gulf, more grim than death, across which there is no reaching. They learn what real loss is by learning that the loss which has to do with shrouds, coffins and the calm finality of soft earth falling is preferable.

To those I would speak and say; (because I know, I have been there) "Remember, when a soul sails out on that unmarked sea called Madness they have gained release much greater than your loss—and more important. Though the need which brought it cannot well be known by those who have not felt it. For what the sane call 'ruin'—because they do not know—those who have experienced what I am speaking of, know the wild hysteria of Madness means salvation. Release. Escape. Salvation from a much greater pain than the stark pain of Madness. Escape—from that which could not be endured. And that is why the Madness came. Deliverance: pure, simple, deliverance."

"Madness knows nothing at all of the human fears which hold us. It knows nothing of wrong doing—has no such thing as conscience—no fear of God or Devils. Nothing in this world can stay it when it has claimed its own. The one whom it has chosen has no choice in the matter. They must follow and obey and try with desperate effort to deliver a satisfying performance. It is the force of living, entangled in the meshes of itself. No one can right it, once the threads become entangled in spinning the thing which is itself."

"No phenomenon of nature is so awe inspiring. A typhoon —a Niagara or the ebb and flow of oceans can be caught and held in harness as easily as a deranged mind! Nothing will stay it— there is nothing that can hold it; nothing with the power to deter it when it sweeps out to pursue its destiny through the dim caverns of itself. There is little known about it, and nothing can stop it when the liberation comes. Though truly— whether it is bondage, or undreamed of liberation depends upon whatever one's idea of those things may be. What is bondage? What is freedom? The interpretation of their definitions fills the answer to the riddle of what Madness is; for it contains the complete and entire significance of both. Though I see evidences of the power of Madness, daily—and the grim mystery of it—and have had much closer knowledge than that. I have felt it sweep me and take me—where—I do not know, (all the way through Hell, and far, far on the other side; and give me keener sense of feeling that the dull edge of reason has)—still, I have no way of telling about the things experienced on that weird journey."

At least I have learned this: nothing is as terrible when it is actually happening to us as when we are dreading, fearing and anticipating it. When and if the thing we fear comes upon us— if it is worth the fear we have expended, we are so enveloped and enmeshed in it we do not have time to worry about it. Worry is the substance which fills vacuity. When we are faced with grim reality we do not spend much time on hypothetical cases.

It is the fear we build in our minds which gives a thing the power to cause us greater pain.

Even Madness—which has been the particular thing I have fled most of my life, was not so terrible when it actually overtook me as it was in all the years during which I tried to escape it. Though to be perfectly frank in the matter I must admit I have been spared the greater pain because some force which seemed at the time to be outside myself protected me. I do not understand it—and if the psychologists who study such odd quirks of personality are able to explain it—they can do more than I.

Only maniacs murder those whom they love. I don't have that on my conscience because some power prevented the blow from falling. Some power outside myself. I had picked up a hammer and aimed it with murderous intent and was filled with a fierce exultation because I felt as powerful as Sampson.

But a curious thing happened. Mid-way in its swing my arm was stopped as though another hand caught it; and I saw it descend to the table, gently; suspendedly, as though it were floating. I watched my fingers relax their murderous grasp on the weapon. Relax slowly, gently in an uncurling sort of a movement with no volition on my part.

It was the surprise at seeing this happen which brought me somewhat to my senses—and I turned and went from the presence of the loved one whom I had so nearly murdered. And though the rest of my body still felt a wild agitation—the hand which had held it was steady and poised and there was an odd tingling sensation extending to my shoulder. I make no attempt to explain it—that is just the way it happened. The next hour was a gethsemane I wish I could forget. It found me on my way to the court house to ask a sanity hearing. They found me insane and sent me here under guard. Perhaps that would have been the end of the story if I could have stopped all thinking—but that is not such a simple matter.

I did get along very well until a letter came from my mother. It was really a lovely letter, asking to come and see me. For no reason at all I felt such a rebellion and bitterness fill me that it rose like a gorge and choked me. I could not reason around it, but there was no reason for it. I hated myself for the monster I was—for repaying all the years of her "love" and all the things she had given me in such cruel coin.

I thought of the thousand ways I loved her and would not admit the hatred I felt had any right to be here because I knew it was obscene and evil.

I felt a pity for her that seemed to be cutting my heart out; I thought of myself—and wondered which of the two was the most pitiable. I thought, how much better had she not prayed for a child—than to have borne me—a Frankenstein monster. But since she had—and it had been locked away where such creatures belong—why should she insist on such a grim resurrection.

Why—Why couldn't she let me lie quietly dead, and mourn me as having departed. I wanted to tear myself limb from limb —to give voice to my frustration with shrieking. But I held it down to soft tears and slipped away from the others into one of the side-rooms. One of the patients passing slipped up behind me and I suppose thinking to cheer me asked why I laughed and what was so funny! I whirled on her in my madness; but held myself back from attacking—because she had done me no wrong. So I went instead to the nurse and said—"Tie me."

She did not tie me down, but locked me away in one of the side-rooms kept for the purpose, first removing all things with which I might injure myself as I'm marked on the chart "suicidal."

Even then she could not remove the thing which was doing the greater injury. It did not lay in her power as it was my own soul within me. The thoughts I had were not "thinking," only the madness of "feeling." A small part of my brain was still able to think with a little logic; and it kept telling me, No, No, No,—the thing upon me was wicked and evil and I must resist it. I tried to, but it seemed I had knowledge only of nameless frustration, rising and tossing in great evil breakers within me. And I was frightened.

A doctor came in and looked at me wonderingly. I lay fighting tears I did not dare shed because they would release that other thing—Madness.

He asked me, "What is the matter?" I could not tell him because I did not know; and I asked him to tell me, if he could.

He tried to; using words so long and high sounding I did not know their meaning.

He laughingly said, "There is nothing wrong with you except you've read too much Freud."

This seemed like a mockery, for to my certain knowledge I had never read a line he wrote.

So I told him: "Whatever the trouble is, you are wrong in trying to make a connection where there could not possibly be one. To me, Freud is only a name, there is no logic in trying to trace my trouble to his door."

But he calmly insisted: "Such is the case, even though you will not admit it."

I did not try to argue—even though at a time of less pain I would have resented the imputation I was lying. Whatever other faults I may have, at least, I tried to be truthful.

Then—as though it ended the problem and left nothing more

to be solved, he said: "You are too egotistical." I could have laughed in his face at the smug wisdom. Of course it was true! Of that there could be no denial. But instead of the end—it was just the beginning of trouble.

I could feel his surprise when I did not contest his assertion. He looked at me oddly when I said: "None knows it better than I, there is entirely too much of me to live with. Since there is —what can I do to hew my gross and unseemly proportions down to a normal size?"

"Think about others," he answered.

That was more mockery, I could not think around the pain raging within me.

He flattered the extent of my knowledge by using terms and phrases at whose meaning I could only guess; then would up with a statement which seemed like sarcasm: "But you know as much about all that as I do."

Whether or not he meant it for mockery, I have no way of knowing; it seemed then like cruel and ironic humor. Something broke in a flood within me—and shook me to the foundation as words poured out in a torrent.

I told him that whether or not he was jesting, I had no knowledge to combat the condition. That my thinking for others could not go beyond a concern for their safety. That I would be as fair as a snake and not strike without warning. I told him I was going mad—and asked him for God's sake to help me if he could. And the thing was lashing within me as I felt the walls of my whole structure crumbling.

Then he said, "I will. I will help you." His face did not seem so smug then; and I thanked him. So hope came again; the part of my mind that could not consent to dissolution, took courage and stood like a rock through that crisis.

He turned to the nurse and said, "Send her to the hydro within thirty minutes."

As the nurse brought me down she seemed very kindly and reassuring. She spoke most encouragingly. She was so accustomed to seeing the patients hang back and rebel in fear of the hydro, she thought that I, too, would resent it. For to come to this place is to be sent to the very bottom of Limbo. It is about the same as stepping off the world altogether. But she did not know how I felt—how gladly I would have gone into Hell to escape the horror stalking me. So I laughed and laid my hand on her arm and thanked her. We were alone on the stairway—and an odd illusion, most pleasant to feel, seemed to fill me.

All the pain I had fell away—leaving only a vacuum. I could feel the rustling whiteness of her starched nurse's skirt. Her small shapely hand resting on my arm seemed ever so lovely as we walked through a bright cube of sunlight streaming through a window.

So I took my place among those in the hydro. The nurses were making ready to give me a "pack"—for that was the doctor's instructions. They told me to strip; one of them stood by to help me. As the patients looked on one of them shrieked and cursed at me.

When I stood there with my great body naked before them, the one who was helping said to the other, "My God! She's a big one. She seems quiet—do you think we ought to tie her?"

"I don't believe so. The doctor said she would ask for a jacket."

The other one laughed and said she did not believe it—she had yet to see a patient ask to be tied. I wondered if I were a freak, even in an insane asylum—but it did not matter.

The first one said, "All right, Big 'Un—we'll try it."

I smiled down at her, for she seemed matter-of-fact and

friendly—and I liked her. Then she talked to me and teased me about what a "case" the doctor had on me, and that he had made a special trip back to the hydro to give instructions about how to treat me. That I was to be "packed" on a mattress, imagine!—when there was not one in the place not being used; and she had got the idea from hearing him talk that I was a priceless and delicate piece of machinery. Then I had turned out to be nothing but a skinned horse! Well, there was no accounting for doctors!

I had a "pack" and ever since that experience the colloquialism, "wet blanket" has assumed gigantic powers of expression.

I was removed from the "pack" at the time the doctor had given. That afternoon he stopped on his round of inspection to ask if it had helped me. I told him it had and offered my hand as I thanked him.

He took my hand; saying gravely, "I am glad," and moved on to the next patient.

So I became one among those in the hydro and lived with the wildly demented—and life flowed on in a shallow and meaningless channel which in no way could be called living. I dared not think with more than one lobe of my brain—a great numbness covered the others. I moved like a machine designed to perform only the mechanics of living. It was good to have it so. The walls of my prison and the heavy barred windows seemed like a massive break-water between me and the responsibility of living. Instead of resenting my fate, I accepted it as something that had to be—scarcely resenting the necessity. Mechanically I fell into step with life as it moved in the hydro. I worked along at whatever had to be done, bathing and feeding the others, and doing other things—tasks done only in an insane asylum.

The next day another of the doctors came through the hydro. (He gave me the only examination thus far given). Asking me questions and writing down answers, tickling the soles of my feet and banging my knee caps with a rubber mallet to test the nervous reflexes. I do not know what he found out about me—but he had been very kindly. I had none of that "something in a test-tube feeling" as he talked to me. He brought two others of his profession down to the hydro and stopped at the table where I was trying to write a letter to my mother. One that would not be too far from the truth, and yet give her some comfort.

He spoke to the doctors and said he wanted them to meet a "Patient who is psychoanalyzing herself—and doing a good job of it."

He laid his hand on my shoulder and looked into my face, very kindly—and at his touch something inside me seemed to dissolve. Because I felt his great kindness I could hardly keep the tears from showing. I caught his hand—before I thought how the gesture might look to those who were watching. I could not speak the words I wanted to say, the tears were too near the surface; but he waited.

I said, "I am sorry I cannot do it because I cannot make heads or tails of the trouble. There is nothing I have been able to dig out which has enough bearing to be of any importance, it seems the best thing for me to do is to give it up altogether. Just throw up my hands and sink."

He just lifted my other hand ever so gently and looked into my face, very gravely.

"Look at me," he said, and I did. His eyes seemed to be turning my features over—hunting for something.

"No!—You are not going to throw your hands up and sink.

You are going to fight this thing through 'till you come out on the other side. Don't give up! You can do it. You will do it—it means an awful lot to me to see you do it. Means much more than you think."

Something in the calm force of his suggestion made it more than a suggestion. It was like a line cast to one drowning. I felt the quiet force of the man himself and felt the words as he spoke them settle into my soul. He had charged them with faith, hope and courage before he sent them.

Before he came I had been in a quagmire with nothing to stand upon but the vast treacherous sucking of despondency beneath my feet. In his kindness he had stooped and placed the firm footing of hope once again beneath me.

I felt my soul come alive and set immediately to rebuilding the walls which had crumbled. He looked and knew it had started. In that moment I became his daughter, for he had begat new life within me, that which had been dead. I saw his eyes mist over with tears. A soul cannot do the thing he had done for me and remain untouched with a benediction.

A fierce determination came to me—born of new hope and courage; and I made a resolve that no matter how greatly I might be tempted to think with a warped crookedness—I would resist it; would hold it down and repel it. And having always before me and with me, so that there was no escaping it, the constant example of these others who had failed and been overcome by their Madness. This example furnished me daily with fresh determination.

So I went about with new courage; and though I could feel the Madness of others sweeping and swirling about me, at times like the rushing of many waters, I stayed firmly grounded on the rock of my self control—and their Madness seemed not to touch me. I had taken up arms again in the battle and vowed that I would not be defeated; that great hulking monster, insanity, should not come out and possess me.

The thing grew the larger because of my determined suppression; for I walked very softly and lived very shallowly, never daring to admit to myself I could not control it. It was there in my mind like a great deformity, but my pride and the great egotism within me, and the terrible fear I had of its triumph made me walk uprightly. I was able to hold it and compel it to keep silent so no one but myself knew just how ugly it was —and they called my fear of it a foolish and senseless phobia.

A loneliness seized me—the like of which I had never known. I wanted something—what I did not know. I felt the stark madness of others beating around me—and I could not endure it.

I felt like a soul cast out of the world. I could not live with those I loved, because of the horror of Madness stalking me.

I could not be accepted among those who are sane because of the thing which marked me as "different." Yet I could not take my place among those who are not until the moorings holding me are broken. I stood amazed at the nakedness and loneliness of living. Yet I felt cords binding me that were closer than my own thoughts of my husband and mother. Something gave way within me. I have no way of telling what it was—except to call its name Madness. Anything that makes a soul feel as I felt at that moment is Madness.

I thought of the man I had married. I remembered the funereal feeling in the long drive up here—and I remembered the tight, stricken look on his face as he told me good-bye—not daring to kiss me. I thought of the years we lived together.

It all broke in a flood around me—everything out of the past was suddenly there in the present. Such a nostalgia came with my thinking I actually felt in my nostrils the dew-laden fragrance of honeysuckle under our window and I heard the sigh and rustle of the leaves in the maple moving the moonlight about in a toss of silvery motion. In that moment my thinking ceased to be thinking and became naked feeling.

I lived again all the things that were passed. I felt the swing of a paint-brush as I had used it in working, and remembered the pride I had felt in the room thus redecorated. I remembered our table and one meal in particular, how glad I had been, how much I had had to enjoy as I sat at the foot and watched him serve our guests. He used my "birthday silver," for which he had saved so long.

I thought of my mother, probably staring outside as I was, seeing nothing. In that moment I knew nothing would ever be different for any of us. She would sit somewhere waiting death and I would sit in the madhouse waiting madness, and the sooner it came for each of us, the better. So the monster was out and the ghost of some old berserker ancestor rose up within me and suggested that I could do something about it, and the fierce hatred exulted that it had possessed itself of a massive and powerful body. And the thing that was in me was not I at all—but another—and I knew that no power on earth but a strait-jacket could hold her.

So I went to the nurse and said, "Tie me."

The voice that asked was not mine; my voice has been called pleasant—but that voice was so flat and hollow it had neither color nor tone. But the nurse was so stupid she mistook the whole meaning and because I displayed no agitation she sent me back to bed. The patient next to me was tied down and raving—and the thought kept persisting, insisting, demanding action. I dared not obey the criminal urge I felt. So I went a second time to the nurse and asked for a jacket. This time the two of them seized and marched me back to my bed. I went ever so gladly—for I thought they meant to tie me. But no. They were going to make me control that which there is no holding. I had controlled it for years, but knew now it was beyond me. I still have an empty, sick feeling when I think of the things which so nearly happened in the hydro that day.

There was still some vestige of fairness left in me. I knew such thoughts as came to me were maniacal; knew I could not resist them for long. So I went a third time to the nurse, but she made a great point of ignoring me. I stood over her with my hands gripping my folded arms tightly because I could not trust them to hang down free at my sides. All my nerves tingled with the madness loose within me—and I thought how pleasant it would be to let my arm swing free and fell her with one mighty blow. I knew I could do it and knew I would if she did not hurry and tie me.

If I live for a thousand years I shall never forget the minutes that followed. She stood there before me with no idea my request was an appeal for help—urgent and necessary. To be put into a jacket I would first have to do something to warrant it—and I had done nothing. But she did not know of that berserk thing in my brain charging and raging. For had I given it the least bit of leeway, even to putting any force in my voice, I could not have held it; nor could any ten of the others have held me. There were not enough people loose in the hydro to have tied me down; and I knew it. But because I still had some decency left, I knew it was up to me to take the initiative. But the nurse could not see any deeper than the deadly calm of the exterior —nor that when my self-control went, it would go out like a flood—and I would be a raging maniac. Something had snapped in my brain and every moment that passed was precious. I had no way of letting her know. I could hardly think or speak. All my energy was being expended to hold the thing down till I could be tied.

I felt all my nerves tingling; an odd light feeling in my head. The force of the impulses charging out of my brain were actually swaying my body. For one split second I had the feeling I had stepped out of my body and was standing there watching. In that short space of time I felt myself praying a desperate prayer as a helpless third person. I looked on the person I knew was myself—and knew I had never seen her. She seemed bigger than any human I ever saw. So deadly and menacing that I felt a nausea of fear and prayed to God to make the nurse hurry!

When the nurse finally took notice of me towering over her she was thoroughly angered because I had not obeyed. I saw the blood flush in her face and heard her voice rising in anger as she spat out, "Go back to your bed. I am not going to tie you."

As I answered my voice was so flat and hollow it seemed to be coming from a great distance. I had the sensation that the whole thing was unreal. I recall having a similar feeling one time as I went under ether. I could not speak a straight-forward sentence—just two or three hollow words with short pauses between them.

I finally managed to say, "I am not going back until you tie me. If anybody has to be hurt it is going to be you. I do not mean to leave you. I have tried to be fair in the matter and if there is to be any consequences—you are the one to whom they will happen, not those helpless people in the dormitory."

She lashed out at me saying, "If you want to fight come right ahead. I will enjoy nothing more than for you to try to fight me."

I knew the deadly woman who stood in the body I had called mine would stop nowhere short of destruction. She should have had sense enough to know it too. Also, that there were not enough of them to have put me into a jacket against my will. With all the strength I had, I tried to hold on to that which was leaving. I held myself so tightly my fingers left raw gashes upon my arms as they gripped and tore them. So she tied me—and did not know the arms that seemed so willing to slip into the jacket were being forced there with the last ounce of will power I had.

When I was tied down securely and could relax my hold upon myself all my shame flowed out in a wild flood of tears. They were partly tears of vexation that I should have been such a coward. That I had not had the courage to do the things I had such an urge to do—but more, they were tears of relief that I had not done them. Mostly, they were tears of rage and confusion at the necessity for the whole unspeakable thing.

The doctor came in and spoke to me, but I did not care what he said; it did not matter. He chided and ridiculed me for giving up so easily—and that did not matter. I was a soul stretched on a rack in a hell very far removed from all ordinary living. The opinions of those whom I had left did not reach through to me—I was too far away. And I do not know whether I was courteous or rude to him. As far as I was concerned his significance had ceased. I lay stretched in the humiliation of the thing which had happened, thoughts of my mother came to me and something she had often said lashed again across my memory.

I heard her voice, filled with cruelty, sneering, "You poor ungodly thing."

Then I saw her eyes and I knew they were at that moment filled with unspeakable anguish at the thing which had overtaken her daughter. And that I had given her such pain because

I had not fulfilled all the beautiful things she had planned for me.

I wondered if she were having any delight in knowing that at least I had fulfilled the contempt she felt for me when I had failed.

I hated her with a fierceness I could not control—had I wanted to. It raged through me with such intensity it seemed I had lived up to a great destiny in fulfilling that much of her expectations. I shrieked out, before I realized there was no one to take the message; that I wanted her to know before she died of old age that at least one seed she had planted in my very babyhood had taken root and grown; that as she had never been able to see anything but failure in her other efforts, I wanted her to take great pleasure in this one—for she had nurtured it more carefully than the other things.

And once the great Madness in me found a voice, there was no stopping it. It rolled out in such a tumult I was amazed at it myself; wondered where it all came from. It seemed obscene and terrible that I should answer in adult language, things said to me in my childhood. Things I had forgotten, until they again began to pour about me in a flood of bitter memories. Even incidents I remembered clearly came back so warped and twisted they seemed like evil changelings.

As I fitted answers to all those unimportant and forgotten childish silences, they lost much of their bitterness. I knew what a foolish, stupid and senseless thing I had done—but it did not matter.

I felt so much better that I had at last found the courage to look and see things as they were (not camouflaging them in the rosy light of a meaning they did not have) that I wanted to shout and sing.

That voice was reason making a last desperate stand—but it was just a shadow and had no power to check the things I was feeling. Still it held me silent for a few short minutes and forced me to consider the thing I knew was happening to me. It brought across my consciousness the recent memory of two patients who had wasted all their life in raving and whom death had overtaken.

Even that memory could not check the flow of thoughts within me and I had to give expression to them somehow. They were greater than my reason and knew nothing of the fear of dying or doing wrong.

All my human fear of pain and death and loss of reason was drowned in wild exultation. I stood upon the brink of everything I had ever feared and knew it did not matter how far into any of them I fell. I knew I was falling and that wild thing within me stood erect and laughed peals of laughter not good to hear. It made my own flesh creep and crawl to hear it because that laughter was never mine—but something wild and terrible.

But even as I fell into the pit yawning beneath me I sent a prayer up to God asking Him, if he had any power in the situation, to please keep my raving from filling my mouth with the crawling and slimy obscenities that I had, without exception, heard the others give voice to when Madness overcame them.

So the last connected and coherent thing in my thinking gave way—and the Madness filling me rejoiced. Because at last there was nothing to stay it, it shouted and exulted with a noise that tore my throat out, charging through me till it nearly dragged the life out of me. Part of my mind stood there and took in the whole situation, yet could do nothing about it. The thing that was raging did not seem wrong to me then—but the rightest thing in the world—a magnificent accomplishment.

The doctor, thinking to quiet me, ordered a hypodermic of apo morphine, a sick hypo. Then a second one—the hours of sleep which should have followed did not come and as the night wore away, my voice became so hoarse there was no pleasure in hearing it and I thought of the others who were trying to sleep, and something of sternness rose up within me as I remembered how often my sleep had been disturbed because of their raving —so I made the thing which drove me content itself with reciting poetry in a low voice so those who were trying to sleep would not be kept awake by my raving.

As the night wore on past midnight, I thought pretty well of myself for considering the others and letting them sleep if they could.

The first thing I was conscious of next morning was Claw-belly across the aisle, saying in a voice that rolled like thunder out of her, "O, God, O God—O God—O God—I wish I was on a lake this morning!"

That would be nice, I thought and wished I were too. I had forgotten all about that awful woman; for I knew I did not want to be anywhere with her alone and free. I had seen enough of her to know I could not trust her. But before I had time to use any reason or do any thinking—I was suddenly free and on a lake! It was not imagination—but something stronger. Mere imagination, however vivid, cannot transport a person tied down hand and foot in an insane asylum to set them free in some far place. I found I was standing somewhere on a pebbly beach at dawn.

I stretched my arms upward and felt the chill morning air around me. I heard the squeak of locks and dip of oars and heard the ripple of water against a boat. I heard the sound of a reel and the small splash the bait made as it hit the water. Mist in little spirals rose from the face of the water, and here and there fish splashed the surface and started widening ripples that chased each other to the edge, losing themselves in the coarse grass growing along the shore.

I felt the crunch of pebbles under my feet in walking, and saw a small frog stretch its legs in a disappearing streak as it took to the water. Rising out of the pungent odor of the dawn was the sharper odor of woodsmoke, and the smell of bacon frying. The willows on the other bank came out in clearer view as they absorbed daylight, and presently they were a soft fluff of color against the darker trees behind them. A blackbird whistled near me and further back a bluejay answered—sharply. I had never seen a dawn so lovely. For I had never been on a lake before which did not exist—nor had I ever experienced a dawn that had not reached me through my dull sense organs —and this was something different—so poignant and perfect it was an ecstasy.

Delusion—is the name the doctors give such happenings.

I knew that awful woman was at the bottom of it—but if she were able to transport me to such a pleasant place, and give me keener eyes and sense of feeling than the dull prosaic thing called sanity—which I had fought so hard to keep—then I had lost but little; and the loss was not worth grieving over.

There was such rest and freedom in floating in the current of my thoughts without the struggle of forcing my thinking to continue in the channels I had been taught were right! So I let them run wild and free and made no effort to think of anything. All the things I had striven for, during a whole lifetime of fierce wanting, fell so far away from me I did not know I had ever suffered disappointment—or unrest—or fear.

As singing is the natural, spontaneous expression of freedom, I felt an urge to sing—for I was free. And I did sing—song after song. Nothing mattered. As one of the patients up on the ward had said: "I was enjoying my insanity."

The nurses came, loosened and led me away from my bed. I did not try to resist them—there was nothing in the world worth struggling for. But when I saw where they were taking me, I laughed and laughed. They had led me to the side-room for solitary confinement. There on the bed was a brand new strait-jacket—the biggest and longest I had ever seen. It was so stiff it stood up and held its shape like a suit of armor. It was as strong as sheet iron. And there was no shame or rebellion at the sight of it—but only something that was ludicrously funny. I slipped into it and laughed as they tied the straps to the bed-rail.

Presently the doctor came in to see me. His face was grave and so concerned I laughed again and tried to tell him I had known this was happening—but that I had been wrong in thinking it mattered. But I was talking across the great distance separating us and I never could get him to see the humor I saw in the situation. He asked the nurse what the sick hypos had done for me and she answered, "Nothing."

I told him she was entirely mistaken—"the first one made me so sick I feared I was dying—and the second one made me so much sicker I feared I wasn't."

He laughed at that and asked me if I wanted another.

I answered, "while I do not greatly desire it—if you want to do something for me and that is all you can think of, send it along. I only asked for a strait-jacket when I felt myself going."

I remembered the two I had seen die in their raving, and others whose Madness had robbed them of everything which made life valuable. But none of the things I recalled had sufficient meaning to make me take up arms again in the conflict. I speculated as to whether I could control it again if I wanted to badly enough, and thought perhaps I could—but more likely I couldn't. I recalled numerous instances when my position as mistress of myself had been very doubtful, and laughed again at the memory of the doctor's face as he stood over me. How gravely concerned he seemed after I had ceased caring.

I wondered what had come over me to make me lose interest in the thing that had mattered so keenly—and I could not recall a single reason why I should have cared in the first place. As I lay there thinking, I suddenly discovered my thoughts were not thoughts—silent and secret—but words, which I was shouting! I could no more shut off the flow of words through my mouth than I could stop the flow of thoughts through my brain. It seemed so unnatural that fresh panic seized me and I was surprised to hear a shriek from my throat at the moment I felt the fear grip me.

I flung out a challenge to the forces wrestling and told them to go to it—that henceforth, I was out of the picture. If the thing that was I was of sufficient importance to be the scene of such conflict—to the victor would belong the spoils. The idea came that if the present rate were continued, it was more than likely the spoils would be so thoroughly ruined the thing over which they were fighting would be of no value to either.

Perfectly good nerves began to snap here and there. There was a radiator directly over my bed, suspended from the ceiling. As I looked at it, it would fade from sight and instead of the ceiling I would be looking through grey, limitless vistas of empty space. Then the radiator would come back into view to fade again.

The endless siege and counter-siege was using up my resources in a prodigal holocaust. Some more nerves snapped in my eye. I saw a great bat flitting in and out behind the radiator, whenever the radiator stayed in view. It was real, though I knew a humming-bird could not get in through the grates at the windows. But the bat was there plainly; near enough to see the point of his wings and feel the shadow he cast, move across me.

Presently, over in the corner I saw a creature about two feet tall jumping up and down. He looked like pictures I had seen of imps and seemed in high glee. I was not afraid of him—he tickled me and I asked the little squirt what he wanted and what he was laughing at. But he disappeared and that made me mad. I never did like wishy-washy will-of-the-wisp things. I looked up and the radiator was gone again—but the bat was circling back and forth where it had been. Another irony struck me. Here I was, a respectable woman who had eschewed liquor all my life—pretty far along in a bad case of delirium tremens.

Presently, I began to tire of lying in one position. I felt the free swing of my arms as I flung them back over my head. I felt the cool bed-rails against them and felt the grasp of my fingers in each hand as I clasped them. That was the eeriest sensation of all—knowing my hands were tied securely in a strait-jacket, yet feeling them free and flung back over my head!

By the morning of the third day I was far away in the ethereal heights of ecstasy.

The doctor came in, looked at me and asked, "How do you feel?"

"Angelic as a fat cherub," I replied.

By the morning of the fourth day I had settled down into

something of the person I still am to this day. The doctor again asked me how I felt.

I answered, "Much too good to be myself."

The fifth morning they took me out of the jacket. I had been wringing wet with perspiration most of the time during those five days and nights and the odor, (stench is the word), which assailed me when that jacket was loosened, was asphyxiating. Truly, something had died, and was decomposing! There was a timbre to the odor of that perspiration which was totally unfamiliar. Even the sweat glands had become a voice in that conflict. My hands were filled with a heavy glutinous substance. Every nerve and fibre in my whole body registered the effect of what I had been through. My whole chemistry was changed. Truly I was a different person.

I have not used fantastic expressions in trying to tell about the experience, but never, if I were able to give a word by word, play by play, account of what happened, would it show the real significance of what transpired—any more than an X-ray picture of an aching tooth is a photograph of the pain.

After a bath, (or perhaps it was a baptism) I felt cleansed and pure. My soul exalted within me. Somehow or other I knew I had left the clown, the shrieks and the delusions behind me. I looked back at the immense expanse of the jacket. There it lay as I had left it. It still held the shape of my body. A perspiration soaked, evil smelling coffin for my madness. Truly I wanted to bury it with great ceremony but without regrets. I left it there with the feeling it contained the stripped down skeleton of a warped and twisted soul.

Suddenly the answer came to me in a flash of brilliancy; like a spotlight outlining a featured player. I was a mental misfit. Like an alcoholic who knows he cannot take even one drink or a diabetic who must forever forego any sugar, I knew I must pass up all depressive thinking. I could not swear off forever. Life here is lived hour by hour, so I must adjust my rebuilt and overhauled mind to a leaner mixture.

I found it very simple, so I said to myself, "I just won't think about it this minute. I'll mentally change the subject just this once and let the next hour take care of itself."

"I'm not cured. I'm just on a 'paraldehyde parole.' I will not break it this time. I'll always think about it tomorrow."

As I wandered about the ward I noticed the "Schizo" staring out the window again.

Seating myself beside her I said, "Say, you remember telling me about being a 'Juke' and having two strikes on you?"

She stared at me with a six-ply scowl for a minute; then said, "No, I don't remember telling you about it, but I will."

Then she proceeded to recount her whole horrible history with many details thrown in she had not mentioned before. Told me that her mother had died of a heart attack when she found out her father had given gonorrhea to three of his young daughters. Told me of her high school days when she and some of her fellow students had indulged in debaucheries so vile I could not repeat them if I tried.

She told me of a brother who had been electrocuted at twenty-two for a crime even more heinous than the famous Loeb-Leopold case. I guided our talk into her service in France during the World War and she said:

"Yes, I was a nurse. I had gotten training after I left home. How I financed these three years is nobody's business."

"Financed it," I exclaimed, "you got paid for training, didn't you?"

"Yeah, I got paid for training, a measly fifteen bucks a month. I needed more. Yeah, I got paid, but I already had plenty of training in the things that paid the most."

"How about the other strike you mentioned?" I asked, "what was that?"

"Other strike," she said, "say, you got a memory like an elephant.—And you're supposed to be crazy."

"Yes, I remember now, I've always said I had two strikes since I found out I was a 'Juke.' The other one I knew about all my life."

"It was bad enough, I think, to have it, but being a Juke and the other thing too, is too much. I couldn't stand it. I guess you know that. I'm here. That proves I couldn't stand something, doesn't it?"

I thought she was going off into another spell of melancholia but she just got up, paced around the floor a few times, then came back and said, "Along with being a born harlot I'm also a Gemini. I was born under the sign of the Twins. I always wondered what made me do the things I did."

"I didn't want to be a girl of 'easy virtue.' I often did things I was sorry for a few minutes later. I'd go to Sunday school and feel all sanctified and holy. Maybe on the way home I'd be tempted and give in."

"But Gemini," I said, "that's just an astrological insignia. It may or may not mean anything."

"It meant something to me," said Schizo, "I read several books on astrology. I found the descriptions given of people born between May twenty-second and June twentieth exactly fit me."

"I was two people. On one hand I liked books and poetry and art and music. I liked people. I liked to talk and be witty. I got a great kick out of being the 'life of the party.' I was considered a good conversationalist, was said to have a lot of personality. Gregarious—they call it. And it's fun."

"I liked to dance and sing, liked noise and laughter, I enjoyed the feeling I got when I did some favor for someone. I was a hail-fellow-well-met."

"There's nothing wrong with these things," I interposed, "some of the nicest people I ever knew were Gemini."

"Of course they are nice people," said Schizo. "They could charm an Eskimo out of his igloo. They can talk most anybody into anything."

"But——," she went on, "they are also a curious combination of Dr. Jekyll and Mr. Hyde. They can be so charming, so nice, so honest one minute and then sink to such levels their own mothers wouldn't claim them."

"Look at me. While in France I tended to wounded soldiers hour after hour. I felt noble. I waited on them hand and foot. I talked to them and soothed them. I'm sure I made life—and death—a lot easier for many of them."

"For instance, late one evening I held a young fellow's hand while he breathed his last. Just at sundown I closed his eyes and notified the medical officer of his death. Then I went to my cot and said a prayer for his soul. I also prayed that his mother and the others who loved him would find solace in knowing he died a hero. Yes, I was noble, I was Dr. Jekyll."

"Then I sneaked down into the grounds of the old chateau in which we were billeted and indulged in some things I was ashamed of. Yes, ashamed of. I hadn't wanted to go. I went, enjoyed the things I was ashamed of, swore I'd never do it again. Then went back the next night and not only repeated them but added to them. I had found a young lieutenant who taught me things even us Jukes didn't know. I've often wondered since if maybe he, too, wasn't a Juke."

"I'm lost. I'm an angel—and a devil. I'm a paragon of virtue —and a vassal of vice. I'm an 'honest' crook—and crookedly honest. I would take money from a blind man—and give it to a cripple. One minute I am chaste. The next I'm chasing, eager for the catch. I'm just no damn good."

"I love life—and wish I were dead. I love everybody—and I've never been in love. I'm the least vain person you ever saw,— yet I am a Narcissi. I'm an angel without wings—and I'm a paving block on the broad-gauge highway to hell. 'Neuro-Cycloid-Schizophrenia,' the doctor said. Schizophrenia hell, I'm just no damn good. I'm a 'Gemini Juke.'"

CHAPTER *13*

A WEEK AGO the Farm-woman stood again at the window looking out at the riot of color after an early morning shower.

She was not raving. She did not charge about or curse. Long she stood, silent, a serene expression of contentment on her face. Her eyes showing a glow of knowledge as if she had suddenly acquired all the wisdom of the ages.

An ethereal radiation seemed to cast its glow all about her. I strolled over curiously to see what was happening. She put an arm affectionately about my shoulders and squeezed me to her as she said: "Goodbye, old girl. You and your Shakespeare have helped a lot. You've at least helped my body when no one could do anything for my mind."

Quite surprised at the control she exhibited and the undertone of impending good news her words led me to expect, I said: "Are you leaving? I shall miss you, but maybe I'll see you on the wards upstairs or in the hallway someday. When do you go? I'm so glad for you I could just cry."

"You may see me 'upstairs,'" she answered, "but it won't be on the ward. I'll not go through that door. I'm making a door of my own."

"I told you I wouldn't stay here and listen to those damn doctors and their pretty words. They tell me, 'Yes, you can go home.

Yes, you will soon again hold seeds in your hand and feel the good earth waiting to receive them.' "

Here she held her nose between thumb and forefinger in a derisive disgusted gesture.

"Pretty words, pretty words, seeds, good earth! Yeah, they tell me all those things and then won't even let me have a flower box."

Thinking she was only moody I left her. After awhile she went to her bed and laid down. The strange effulgence continued.

Supper time came and went. The nurses had skipped her lunch and did not disturb her for supper. They did not know what she was thinking. Strangely enough, they would have cared. She had been here so long and was usually so amiable they loved her.

During the night she started raving. She was put into a jacket as soon as the day nurses came on.

Days passed. Her raving continued. Her constant tossing and heaving would have exhausted a less robust person. On the seventh or eighth day she quieted down suddenly. The look in her eyes drew me to her.

I was amazed, as I stood beside her bed, to see her face was not contorted from her ravings. It was smooth and serene. I had the odd feeling her "raving" these past days had been synthetic.

Very quietly, with a calm dignity about her, she said:

"This is the day. I've found out how to do it. I can create pressure myself, greater than 'insanity.' "

As I prepared to remonstrate with her she continued: "It's no use. Don't try to give me any more 'pretty words,' please.

I'm saying goodbye now. Watch me! You may someday want to know how it's done."

Seeing that any attempt to argue with her was worse than useless, I turned away.

As I left her she began to struggle—silently, viciously. The veins on her neck stood out like blue cords against her olive skin. Her eyes became dilated, yet did not lose their rational expression.

Twisting—straining—rolling, she lay there, still silent. She seemed as one wrestling with a python. No one could imagine the terrific effort she put forth, yet she did not seem to be trying to escape the jacket. Rather she was using it to brace her straining against.

Suddenly she let loose a low, moaning roar. No words, no raving, just that hideous, continuous, never-stopping roar. As the night wore on it got louder and louder. The whole place went mad. The monotonous ear shattering roar of the Farm-woman coupled with the shrieks and cursing of the others kept us all awake and cowering from the noise as if from something physical. Howling, shrieking, cursing, roaring. All night it went on. The vibrations of sound it set up in the hydro were horrible. It was like being in the midst of an artillery barrage.

Just when it seemed no eardrum could stand it without shattering, like a wineglass hit with a high C, the Farm-woman set forth a series of high pitched shrieks, yet her roaring did not stop, was not even interrupted. She seemed to have two voices, two sets of vocal cords, one a high-pitched thin, shrill, whistling scream and the other a deep bass low-score-left-key booming. Both of them emitting their infernal, unbearable noises at the same time.

It could only compare to a summer thunderstorm. Black clouds rolled and tumbled across her face. Showers of raindrops ran off her forehead in slow moving beads of sweat.

The olive of her complexion turned the black clouds into the deadly green of an approaching hail storm.

The lightning of her shrieks ripped the air apart and the roaring thunder filled in the vacuum.

As the dawn broke and the sun climbed into view on the window ledge there was a hush. Such a hush was never heard. Of course I'm crazy too, I should know a hush cannot be heard —but this one was. Such sudden quiet was worse than the noise. To be projected from the hell of the raving into the absolute ultimate of tomblike silence required bracing against. It was like a deep sea diver being instantly brought to the surface or like someone walking against the wind who suddenly finds himself in the vacuous center of an exploding tornado. Such an expectant silence is heard only when a famous conductor steps onto the podium and raises his baton.

Not a sound, not even of breathing could be heard. The vibrations rolled around, bouncing off the walls and reverberating into the corners until they died away, but this was not sound—it was feeling.

For this one awful moment of simultaneous silence even the wildest among us stopped raving. I do not know why, perhaps the physicists could measure something and tell. They could have weighed the noise but would have had to slice up the silence.

The Farm-woman rose upright in bed and seemed to stretch forth her arms. True, she was tied, but I was not the only one who thought they saw her do it.

An ecstatic look came over her face as she said, "Yes, I'm ready. I've found the 'door.'"

At that instant the sun broke into full view. As we stood there, transfixed, rooted to our tracks, a tiny bit of vapor seemed to pass from her and dispel itself into the sun.

Was it a bit of early morning mist floating upwards? Was it her last breath condensed by the coolness of the dawning, or—had she "met the messenger"?

She fell back—dead. Two tiny little trickles of blood ran from her nostrils and congealed.

She's gone. "Cerebral hemorrhage," the doctor told us. He wasn't kidding anybody. He should have said "the will to die."

The nurses have come with a hypodermic and a strait-jacket for the beautiful girl who goes naked. She has been standing for an hour howling out a window. Her voice is as indescribable as a voice out of Hell. Nothing I have ever heard is anything like it. Shriek after shriek makes the roots of the hair draw together and the nerves down the spine shudder and quiver.

She is such a beautiful girl—strikingly, startlingly beautiful; and mad as the hatter! Today as I lay on my bed she crawled into my arms and lay there talking to me. I tried to catch the drift of the things she was saying—but could not. Occasionally she'd place her hands against my shoulders and push herself from me, her arms tense and rigid, quivering with the excitement she was feeling. Her back was a beautiful arching curve as she tried to make me look into her eyes. I could not do it, such things are Madness.

I have wrestled and overcome her with massive, brute strength. But today, she held me in the grip of some power akin to mesmerism; I could not send her away—she had chosen me and I could not escape. She had chosen me; and I had to watch her, look at her, be a companion to her; I could not escape her. Nor did I want to. I wanted to see, if I could, the things she saw. I couldn't, though she made me feel them, even though she spoke no words in my ear which made sense. A primeval urge again. Just another "exception" to prove your own rule.

The Skeleton is at another window clutching her fleshless shoulders and shrieking. A new patient is threshing about, cursing and howling. The Camel is snoring. The Field-mouse is grieving.

The Student is standing in the aisle where the nurse left her to help with the Pagan.

The girl at the window eluded their grasp and has slipped to a sitting position, arms thrown upward and head flung backward so her throat is one straight, taut, quivering line.

Claw-belly is laughing and cursing and the Mother who hates to be tied is raving and crying.

The Preacher is lying with a pillow over her head—and I am as crazy as they are. What does my sitting here hanging on to a half chewed pencil amount to? The Student has had no exercise since God knows when—and tonight she is going to dance with me—for no other reason than because I am in the mood to do something crazy—and that is the craziest thing I can think of!

Well—that was that! We danced—and almost got put into jackets! I caught her up and told her I was tired of seeing her stand around like a stick and that whether she liked the idea or not she was going to dance. When we started out, her feet were just dragging as I pushed and pulled her around to the tune of "The Blue Danube."

I suppose we were such a pair as could not be seen outside a bug-house. I had on a long outing gown and she was stark naked. I do not know where anybody got the idea she was a stick! Once she got into the swing of the rhythm she took the lead and all at once began to whirl me about in a maze of steps that I could never have followed if I were sane.

She moved the rhythm up to "Goofus" and by that time my feet had begun to make a slapping sound against the concrete. I could not keep up with her. The nurse heard us, she came running and told us she would tie us both down if we did not stop at once. I put the brakes on so suddenly I nearly fell over my own feet. The Student, with no one pushing or pulling, ran and sprang into her bed. Smiling like an imp back at me, she whirled and buried her face in the pillow.

I had never seen her move before unless someone else pulled or pushed her! And did I get a royal bawling out! I tried to remonstrate that the dance had helped her—and pointed out that she got into bed by herself afterwards. The nurse told me I knew nothing about it and the first thing I knew I would have her raving.

She is lying there yet; turned over again by herself just this minute! And flashed me another of those impish smiles! And I never saw her face change expression before! Tell me that dance did not help her—I know better!

Ho hum—bedtime.

Came the morning—and another miracle! This morning the Student spoke the first words I ever heard pass her lips. We had biscuits for breakfast, she came up to the serving table and stood a moment.

"I want a biscuit."—It was a child's voice—a small voice that has not been used for many long months, but she spoke.

I am so glad I could cry about it! The nurses can think what they like—I still think I had a hand in it—for the first indication of consciousness she has given for months came last night when I dragged her into a dance. If dancing helped her I am glad I did it.

If finding her feet moving to a rhythm which gave her pleasure somehow helped her brain to move to the rhythm of thinking— then I am glad I danced with her. And even if it is all a delusion on my part and if the thing would have happened anyway, dancing or no—it is an odd coincidence that it should come at that moment. And even if it is just a coincidence, it is most pleasant to believe I have brought something of life to another.

She does seem more alive this morning. Her face is alert. There is a vital something about her this morning which has never been there since I first saw her. Nor is she sitting in the haphazard slump that has always characterized her posture previously. I am so glad I wish there was some place to slip off for a good cry about it!

Claw-belly has wriggled out of her jacket and turned the shower on. I do not know why she did not get under it—as hot and sweaty as she gets in a jacket. She turns it on every chance she gets but never gets under it. She has laid back down on her bed and is lying with her eyes closed, listening to the water with a look of beatific contentment on her face. Although she is stinking with streaming perspiration, jackets are a torture when it is hot, she has no imagination to include the things which give comfort to the body. All that's important is to find something to satisfy the pain of her thinking.

The sound of running water must suggest something very lovely to her; she is smiling and has raised her hands above her head to trail them in the sound of the water. She seems very happy, lying there with her eyes closed to further enhance the joy of her thoughts. Her lips are curved in an expression of rapt pleasure. Her long white arms wave slowly as they trail her flowing fingers in the sound of splashing water. She makes no sound herself but lies there listening in enraptured silence. Her pleasure will be short as the nurses now are on their way to tie her poor torn body—and tear the spell of ecstasy from her miserable soul.

They turned the water off abruptly, have caught her feet, tied them and already have the jacket on her. She is howling now and all the pleasure of a few moments ago is gone. Delusions can sometimes be very lovely, but they are made of frail stuff. She is insane. The nurses are sane and that gives them the right to deal with delusions in a most matter-of-fact manner. She was disturbing no one; and I do not see why they could not have left her to her odd pleasure for a little while. True— she is insane.

No sane person could be enraptured simply by trailing their hands in the sound of running water—but she was happy at it till they put a finish to it.

I do not see why they could not allow her a few gallons of water. The state could well have spared it in the face of greater waste. But no. They tied her. And now she is howling and her throat is strained and spreading—to make greater exit for the racket and I feel my own throat closing as I listen to her.

Now she is cursing foully—and I do not blame her. It was such a small thing she wanted but she couldn't have it because she is insane and there is no sense in wanting to trail your fingers in the sound of running water. So howl it out, Claw-belly. They cannot stop that. But personally I would rather see you happy in your delusion, whatever it was—than to hear you raging because you are insane.

/235/

Another of the patients died last night. The woman who had the high temperature. The little new-born baby is bereft of its mad mother and that is that. The very air around here is filled with tragedy of one kind or another, and the individual atoms bearing their full quota of pain must continue with the burden till their release also comes. The knowledge that it is finished for one of the number, does not excite even passing, casual interest. She no longer rolls her head lamenting about "seeing her mistake." Her people went their way without her—and the news of her death probably will not reach them until too late to attend her burial.

There will be two new ones sent to take her place—for there is something insatiable in the great maw of dementia. It claims its victims faster than the state can house and treat them. From the increasing numbers it seems as though the whole world is going mad. Shakespeare and I kept writing in an effort to escape it. It seems as though, now, perhaps we shall make the grade.

I have sat through floods of raving and built a barrier—a break-water of small black words around me. Day by day I've sat here in it and wrote about it—for there was nothing else in all this world to do. The nurse just came and told me that tonight I am being transferred again to the ward upstairs; to the "best" ward. There to take up living in a semi-civilized state.

I must make the most of my pencil while I still have it; and Shakespeare, with me. For I cannot take him to that "semi-civilized purgatory" upstairs. And there is the Pagan, young, lovely, with an exotic quality of beauty so real, so poignant, so altogether different I do not know how—with only the blunt point of a lead pencil and the inadequate words I have at my command, to get a likeness of her onto paper. A pencil and common-place words. With these I cannot depict the noonday brightness of the highlights in her loveliness or shade the shadows of midnight blackness in the tragic abyss which envelops her!

THE PAGAN

Whose hair has the shimmer of sunlight on sand
   With riffles of dust for the shadows
Whose limbs are nimble and lithe, and formed like the figures
      in "Day-break."
Whose eyes are colored with cobalt, wide-set and wondering
      Widening now and anon with a look that on-looking
         eyes,
Beholding
      Look hastily elsewhere—and try to forget what,
Once seen, is remembered forever.
Ecstasy—Madness
      The beauty and majesty of it.
The despair of a soul that has felt what cannot be thought;
   And once feeling; thinks never again.
Shallow thoughts to share with another.

One evening at sundown she sat on the floor by a window
In a pattern of light, cross-checked by the bars that confined
         her,
Her gown cast aside, completely discarded; disclosing
      The smooth white flesh of her body
      A transparent column of beauty
Through which her blood raced, red-flowing and rapid,
Revealing the tension of nerves, tightly stretched and too
         charged
With vibrantly humming emotion
For earthly expression or speech—'til her Madness tran-
      scended

All method and mode of expression.
And wrought for itself
    A vehicle. A cry! Like the shriek of the damned
        Only lovely and lengthening—lengthening—ever rose
            higher in pitch—ever higher
        'Til it pierced through the high-vaulted heavens.
Perhaps God, Who created her, can understand,
    But to us who looked on
        She was just
    An insane daughter of man.

Shakespeare is worn out and eager to get out of this racket and slip back to his quiet grave in far England. All things end sometime or other—and the nurse will come shortly to take me upstairs. So goodbye William. You were one grand delusion! If you had not come to me, perchance this transfer would have been to a place still lower in this limbo—instead of one step upward. I shall hate to lose you—but I cannot take you with me because delusions of grandeur are not allowed upstairs. Goodbye William. I am most grateful to you for coming to me. Goodbye. And may long years of peace and rest attend you in your quiet English grave.

Commencement